PLANT BASED

CKD STAGE 5

COOKBOOK

Healthy and Delicious Low Sodium, Low Phosphorus and Low Potassium Recipes to Reverse Chronic Kidney Disease

David T. Salcedo

HOW TO USE THIS COOKBOOK

Understand Your Dietary Needs

Before digging into the cookbook, make sure you understand your individual dietary restrictions and demands for CKD Stage 5. This could include limits on potassium, phosphorus, and salt intake. Consult your healthcare team or a qualified dietician to determine your specific needs.

Review the Book

Begin by reading the aspect of the book that briefly explains the disease. This will give you important background knowledge on the fundamentals of a plant-based diet designed for CKD Stage 5. Pay close attention to any suggestions, instructions, or recommendations provided to improve your cooking experience.

Explore the Table of Contents

Take time to read the table of contents. This will provide an overview of the recipes included in the cookbook. Identify categories or specific recipes that correspond to your interests and nutritional needs. The cookbook is designed so that you can easily find recipes that meet your specific needs.

Select Recipes Based on Preferences and Requirements:

Choose dishes that suit your nutritional demands and personal tastes. The cookbook provides a variety of options, whether you want a refreshing beverage, a robust main course, or a fulfilling snack. Make a note of any specific substances that require special care, such as low-potassium or low-phosphorus alternatives.

Gather Ingredients and Follow Instructions

Once you've decided on a dish, thoroughly study the ingredients and instructions. Gather all the necessary components, taking care to measure them precisely. Follow the step-by-step instructions provided, and don't be afraid to change the recipes to suit your tastes while staying within your dietary limits.

TABLE OF CONTENTS

INTRODUCTION

Olivia, a vibrant woman, resided in a tiny town nestled between rolling hills and lovely lakes when she was diagnosed with Chronic Kidney Disease (CKD) Stage 5. Determined to regain control of her health, she began on a life-changing journey using the healing power of a plant-based diet.

Olivia's journey began with a diagnosis that made her feel overwhelmed and concerned about the future. With the awareness that her dietary choices could have a big impact on her health, she chose to investigate the advantages of a plant-based lifestyle.

Olivia discovered, via research and consultation with healthcare professionals, that a plant-based diet could help manage the course of CKD. She observed that plant-based diets are naturally lower in potassium and phosphorus, which are important factors for those with severe renal disease. Olivia was intrigued by the possible health benefits of plant-based eating and eagerly embraced the concept.

Her kitchen became a hotbed for innovation and exploration. Olivia sourced a range of colorful fruits, vegetables, legumes, and nutritious grains, carefully choosing foods that met her renal dietary requirements. She learned to replace animal proteins with plant-based alternatives high in critical elements, laying the groundwork for kidney-friendly meals.

Breakfasts became lively affairs, with quinoa bowls garnished with fresh berries and almonds, providing a nutrient-dense start to the day. Olivia's lunches were robust salads brimming with leafy greens, lentils, and a variety of bright veggies, creating a symphony of flavors and kidney-friendly nutrients.

Olivia experimented with recipes such as roasted vegetable stir-fries and sweet potato and black bean casseroles to expand her knowledge of plant-based proteins for dinner. She learnt how to balance flavors, textures, and nutritional values while adhering to her dietary constraints.

Snacks were no longer an afterthought; cucumber and hummus bites, as well as homemade trail mix, became filling options to fulfill lunchtime appetites without jeopardizing her renal health. Desserts were transformed into guilt-free indulgences, with avocado chocolate mousse and banana-oat cookies becoming her go-to sweets.

Olivia's experience continued beyond the kitchen. Armed with a meal planner, she practiced attentive portion control and incorporated regular exercise into her routine, recognizing that a comprehensive strategy was essential for treating CKD. She embraced stress-relieving hobbies and valued quality sleep to improve her general well-being.

Olivia's plant-based lifestyle has a long-term effect on her health. Regular checkups revealed improved kidney function, and she felt more energized and focused. Olivia's journey was not without hurdles, but her dedication to her health and the support of a plant-based diet enabled her to face CKD Stage 5 with fortitude and positivity.

Olivia's health fluctuated with the changing seasons in her little village. Her experience became an inspiration to others experiencing similar issues, indicating that a plant-based diet might be a powerful ally in controlling Chronic Kidney Disease and supporting overall heath.

CHRONIC KIDNEY DISEASE (CKD) STAGE 5

CKD Stage 5, commonly known as End-Stage Renal Disease (ESRD), is the most severe stage of chronic kidney disease, in which the kidneys have almost completely lost function. Individuals with Stage 5 CKD typically require renal replacement therapy, such as dialysis or a kidney transplant, to survive.

Causes of CKD Stage 5

1. **Diabetes:** Uncontrolled diabetes is a common cause since high blood sugar levels can harm the kidneys over time.

2. **Hypertension (High Blood Pressure):** Chronic high blood pressure can cause renal damage and contribute to CKD progression.

3. **Glomerulonephritis:** Inflammation of the kidney's filtering units (glomeruli) can cause irreparable damage.

4. **Polycystic Kidney Disease (PKD):** is a hereditary condition characterized by the development of cysts in the kidneys, resulting in functional deterioration.

5. **Infections and Obstructions:** Recurrent kidney infections or urinary tract obstructions can contribute to the development of chronic kidney disease.

Symptoms of CKD Stage 5

1. **Fatigue:** Fatigue refers to persistent tiredness and weakness.

2. **Fluid Retention:** : Swelling in the legs, ankles, or around the eyes caused by the body's inability to remove extra fluid.

3. **Shortness of Breath:** The accumulation of fluid in the lungs can cause trouble breathing.

4. **Changes in Urination:** Urinary changes include decreased urine flow, black or frothy urine, and increased frequency of urinating.

5. **Nausea and Vomiting:** can be caused by a buildup of waste materials in the bloodstream.

Treatment for CKD Stage 5

1. **Dialysis**

   - **Hemodialysis:** This involves filtering blood outside the body using a machine.

   - **Peritoneal Dialysis:** It uses the abdominal lining to filter waste within the body.

2. **Kidney Transplant**

   - Kidney transplant from a healthy donor, either living or deceased.

Preventive Measures and Lifestyle Changes

1. **Manage Underlying Conditions**

   - Manage blood sugar levels (for diabetes)

   - Optimize blood pressure with drugs and lifestyle modifications.

2. **Adopt a Kidney-Friendly Diet**

   - Limit your salt, potassium, and phosphorus intake.

   - Consider adopting a plant-based diet if appropriate for the individual.

3. **Regular Exercise**

- Improves blood pressure and overall wellness.

4. **Quit Smoking**

- Smoking can damage kidney and cardiovascular health.

5. **Limit Alcohol Intake**

- Excessive alcohol drinking may lead to high blood pressure.

6. **Regular Monitoring**

- Regular check-ups and monitoring of renal function.

THE IMPORTANCE OF A PLANT-BASED DIET FOR CHRONIC KIDNEY DISEASE (CKD) PATIENTS

Chronic Kidney Disease (CKD) is a progressive illness that impairs the kidney's capacity to function properly over time. As CKD progresses, dietary choices become increasingly important in controlling symptoms, delaying progression, and preserving overall health. A plant-based diet has emerged as an effective and well-studied treatment for people with CKD. Here's a thorough examination of the significance of adopting a plant-based diet in the context of CKD:

1. Managing Nutrient Intake

a. Lowering Sodium Content

Plant-based diets, particularly those concentrated on whole foods, typically have lower salt levels. This is crucial for CKD patients, who frequently need to limit their sodium intake to maintain fluid balance and blood pressure.

b. Adjusting Potassium Levels

Plant-based foods often contain less potassium than animal-based ones. Potassium levels must be managed in CKD patients, and a plant-based diet improves control of this mineral.

c. Controlling Phosphorus Intake

Plant-based proteins often contain less phosphorus than animal proteins. This is useful for CKD patients who need to control their phosphorus intake to avoid consequences like bone damage.

2. Supporting Kidney Function

a. Reducing Oxidative Stress

Plant-based diets are high in antioxidants, which can reduce oxidative stress. Oxidative stress can cause kidney damage, while an antioxidant-rich diet may help kidney function.

b. Managing Inflammation

Chronic inflammation is a frequent characteristic of CKD. Plant-based diets, particularly those high in fruits, vegetables, and whole grains, offer anti-inflammatory qualities that may help reduce inflammation linked with kidney disease.

3. Improving Heart Health

a. Lowering Cholesterol Levels

Plant-based diets have been related to reduce cholesterol levels, reducing the risk of cardiovascular problems associated with chronic kidney disease.

b. Regulating Blood Pressure

Hypertension is a common complication of CKD. Plant-based diets, which are known for their beneficial effects on blood pressure, can help regulate this critical part of kidney health.

4. Slowing CKD Progression

a. Preserving Residual Kidney Function

Research suggests that a plant-based diet may decrease the progression of CKD by lowering renal workload and preserving residual kidney function.

b. Enhancing Nutrient Bioavailability

Plant-based diets enhance nutrient bioavailability and absorption, ensuring CKD patients receive important vitamins and minerals for overall health.

5. Weight Management

a. Promoting Healthy Weight

A well-balanced plant-based diet can help manage weight. Maintaining a healthy weight is critical for CKD patients since excess weight can accelerate the progression of renal disease.

6. Psychological and Emotional Well-being

a. Varied and Flavorful Options

Plant-based diets provide CKD patients with a variety of flavor and texture options, leading to better quality of life.

b. Empowering Patients

Adopting a plant-based diet can help CKD patients take charge of their health and feel more empowered.

BASICS OF PLANT-BASED NUTRITION

Plant-based diets have received significant attention and acknowledgment because to its possible health benefits, environmental sustainability, and ethical implications. These diets emphasize plant-based foods while reducing or eliminating animal items. The word "plant-based" is broad and can refer to a variety of approaches, including vegetarianism, veganism, flexitarianism, and the Mediterranean diet. Here's a thorough summary of plant-based diets, including their types, benefits, problems, and critical considerations:

Types of Plant-Based Diets

1. **Vegetarianism**

   - **Lacto-Ovo Vegetarian:** Avoids meat, fish, and poultry but consumes dairy and eggs.

   - **Lacto Vegetarian:** exclude meat, fish, and poultry but include dairy.

   - **Ovo Vegetarian** excludes meat, fish, and poultry, but accepts eggs.

2. **Veganism**

- No form of animal products, such as meat, dairy, eggs, and honey.

3. **Flexitarianism**

- Predominantly plant-based diet with occasional eating of meat and animal products.

4. **Pescatarianism**

- Plant-based, including fish and seafood.

5. **Mediterranean Diet:**

- Emphasizes plant-based meals, whole grains, and healthy fats, with modest amounts of seafood and dairy.

CHALLENGES AND CONSIDERATIONS

1. Nutrient Deficiency

Planning ahead of time is crucial for getting enough critical nutrients like protein, vitamin B12, iron, zinc, and omega-3 fatty acids, which are often lacking in plant-based foods.

2. Protein Sources:

Plant-based protein sources like beans, lentils, tofu, and almonds can help meet amino acid requirements, but it's important to diversify your consumption.

3. Iron Absorption

Plant-based iron (non-heme iron) is less absorbable than iron from animal sources. Consuming vitamin C-rich foods alongside iron-rich plant foods may improve absorption.

4. Social and Cultural Considerations

Adhering to a plant-based diet might be challenging in social situations, cultural contexts, or locations with limited plant-based options.

5. **B12 Supplementation**

Those on strict plant-based diets may need to supplement with vitamin B12, which is predominantly found in animal sources.

IMPORTANT CONSIDERATIONS FOR A BALANCED PLANT-BASED DIET

1. **Diversity of Foods**

Eating a variety of fruits, vegetables, whole grains, legumes, nuts, and seeds provides a diverse range of nutrients.

2. **Fortified Foods**

Use fortified foods or supplements with nutrients found in animal products, such as B12 and vitamin D.

3. **Mindful Planning:**

Planning meals to fulfill nutritional needs and consulting with a trained nutritionist for tailored advice.

4. **Balanced Macronutrients**

Getting the right balance of carbs, proteins, and healthy fats in the diet.

5. **Gradual Transition**

Transitioning to a plant-based diet can be successful with incremental changes that enable the body to adapt.

NUTRITIONAL REQUIREMENTS FOR CHRONIC KIDNEY DISEASE (CKD) STAGE 5

Chronic renal Disease (CKD) Stage 5, also known as End-Stage Renal Disease (ESRD), is the most advanced stage of renal dysfunction, in which the kidneys have nearly completely lost their ability to function. Managing the dietary components of CKD Stage 5 is critical for maintaining general health, managing symptoms, and improving the efficacy of therapies such as dialysis or kidney transplant. Here's an in-depth look at the nutritional requirements for those in CKD Stage 5:

1. Protein Intake

a. Purpose

Protein supports tissue regeneration, immunological function, and muscular mass.

b. Recommendation

Protein requirements vary dependent on age, weight, and health. A moderate protein intake is frequently advised to avoid overloading the kidneys.

c. Sources

Moderate consumption of high-quality protein sources, including lean meats, poultry, fish, eggs, and dairy products. Plant-based proteins, such as beans, lentils, tofu, and grains, can be included.

2. Sodium (Salt) Restriction

a. Purpose

- Lowering sodium intake improves fluid balance and blood pressure regulation.

b. Recommendation

A low-sodium diet is usually recommended. This includes reducing processed foods, avoiding excessive use of table salt, and opting for fresh, natural foods.

3. Potassium Management

a. Purpose

Regulating potassium is crucial for avoiding heart and muscle issues.

b. Recommendation

Monitor your potassium intake. Bananas, oranges, tomatoes, and potatoes are high in potassium and may need to be reduced.

4. Phosphorus Control

a. Purpose

Managing phosphorus levels is critical for preventing bone and cardiovascular issues.

b. Recommendation

Limit foods high in phosphorus, such as dairy, nuts, and some cereals. Phosphorus binders can also be prescribed.

5. Fluid Management

a. Purpose

Maintaining fluid balance can prevent issues like high blood pressure and heart failure.

b. Recommendation

Monitoring fluid intake is crucial. Individuals may need to reduce their fluid intake, which includes water, drinks, and high-water foods.

6. Caloric Requirements

a. Purpose

Adequate calorie intake prevents malnutrition and promotes overall health.

b. Recommendation

Caloric requirements vary depending on age, weight, and activity level. A trained dietician can help you optimize your calorie intake to your specific needs.

7. Vitamin and Mineral Supplementation

a. Purpose

CKD Stage 5 patients may need vitamin and mineral supplements due to limited food options or reduced absorption.

b. Recommendation

Vitamin supplements, including B12, folic acid, and water-soluble vitamins, may be administered.

8. Individualized Meal Planning

a. Purpose

Customized meal plans accommodate nutritional demands and dietary restrictions.

b. Recommendation

Working with a qualified dietitian helps create individualized meal plans based on individual preferences, cultural variables, and nutritional needs.

9. Monitoring Blood Levels

a. Purpose

Regular blood tests monitor nutritional levels and suggest dietary modifications.

b. Recommendation

Regular monitoring of blood parameters, such as electrolytes, minerals, and vitamins, is critical for personalized dietary therapy.

BENEFITS OF PLANT-BASED EATING FOR KIDNEY HEALTH

Adopting a plant-based eating approach has received attention for its potential benefits in maintaining general health, and it is especially important in the context of kidney health. Plant-based diets high in fruits, vegetables, whole grains, legumes, nuts, and seeds have various benefits for those with kidney problems, including chronic kidney disease (CKD). Here's a thorough examination of the advantages of plant-based diets for kidney health:

1. Reduced Sodium Intake

a. Purpose

Plant-based diets typically contain lower sodium levels, leading to improved blood pressure control and reduced fluid retention.

b. Impact on Kidneys

Lowering sodium intake can help manage hypertension, which contributes to kidney damage and disease development.

2. Optimal Blood Pressure Control:

a. Purpose

Plant-based diets can reduce blood pressure.

b. Impact on Kidneys

Optimal blood pressure is essential for preserving renal function. Plant-based diets help regulate blood pressure and may decrease the course of kidney disease.

3. Improved Antioxidant Status:

a. Purpose

Plant-based diets contain antioxidants that reduce oxidative stress.

b. Impact on Kidneys

Oxidative stress is linked to kidney disease. Consuming a range of antioxidant-rich fruits and vegetables may protect the kidneys against oxidative damage.

4. Reduced Inflammation

a. Purpose

Plant-based diets have anti-inflammatory qualities.

b. Impact on Kidneys

Chronic inflammation is linked to renal disease progression. Plant-based diets may help reduce inflammation and improve kidney health.

5. Balanced Protein Intake

a. Purpose

Plant-based proteins are often lower in phosphorus and can be a better option for persons with renal disease.

b. Impact on Kidneys

Managing phosphorus intake is critical in CKD. Plant-based proteins such as beans, lentils, and tofu supply protein without containing too much phosphorus.

6. Heart Health Benefits

a. Purpose

Plant-based diets can improve cardiovascular health.

b. Impact on Kidneys

Cardiac disease frequently coexists with kidney disease. A heart-healthy plant-based diet may minimize the incidence of cardiovascular consequences in those with kidney problems.

7. Improved Glycemic Control

a. Purpose

Plant-based diets promote improved blood sugar control.

b. Impact on Kidneys

Improved glycemic management is especially useful for those with diabetes, which is a leading cause of kidney disease.

8. Healthy Weight Management

a. Purpose

- Plant-based diets help with weight loss and management.

b. Impact on Kidneys

- Maintaining a healthy weight is key to treating renal disease. Plant-based diets may help with weight loss and reduce the stress on the kidneys.

9. Lower Acid Load

a. Purpose

- Plant-based diets often have lower dietary acid load.

b. Impact on Kidneys

- Reducing acid load can lower the risk of metabolic acidosis, which is common in advanced renal disease patients.

10. Alkaline Diet Support

a. Purpose

- Plant-based diets can promote an alkaline environment in the body.

b. Impact on Kidneys

- An alkaline diet may help manage kidney-related problems, but further research is needed.

11. Reduced Phosphorus Intake

a. Purpose

- Plant-based diets are inherently lower in phosphorus compared to animal diets.

b. Impact on Kidneys

- Lowering phosphorus consumption benefits CKD patients by reducing problems associated with high phosphorus levels.

12. Environmental Sustainability

a. Purpose

- Plant-based diets have less environmental impact.

b. Impact on Kidneys

- Sustainable eating choices support general health and well-being.

ESSENTIAL INGREDIENTS AND COOKING TIPS

Building a plant-based pantry for Chronic Kidney Disease (CKD) patients necessitates careful consideration of dietary limits while offering a choice of delectable and nutritious options. CKD patients frequently need to monitor their mineral intake, such as potassium, phosphorus, and salt. A well-stocked plant-based pantry can help people with CKD prepare delicious, kidney-friendly meals. Here's a comprehensive guide to creating a plant-based pantry customized for CKD patients:

1. Whole grains

a. Choices

Includes Quinoa, bulgur, farro, brown rice, and whole wheat pasta.

b. Considerations

Choose whole grains for high fiber content and lasting energy. Rinse grains before cooking to remove excess potassium.

2. Legumes

a. Choices

Lentils, chickpeas, black and white beans.

b. Considerations

Legumes are a great plant-based protein source. Rinse canned types to reduce salt content.

3. Plant-Based Protein

a. Choices

Plant-based protein sources include tofu, tempeh, edamame, and seitan (textured vegetable protein).

b. Considerations

Choose moderate protein consumption and alter quantities to meet individual needs.

4. Nuts and seeds

a. Choices

Nuts and seeds: almonds, walnuts, chia, flax, hemp, and pumpkin.

b. Considerations

Monitor portion sizes for phosphorus content. Nuts and seeds provide healthful lipids and omega-3 fatty acids.

5. Alternatives To Flour

a. Choices:

Use almond, coconut, and oat flour.

b. Considerations

Useful baking alternatives. Adjust quantities based to your dietary limitations.

6. Non-dairy Milk

a. Choices

Almond, rice, oat, or hemp milk are low in potassium and phosphorus.

b. Considerations

Look for fortified options to boost calcium and vitamin D intake.

7. Low Potassium Vegetables

a. Choices

Cucumber, cauliflower, bell peppers, and zucchini.

b. Considerations

To support kidney health, choose veggies with lower potassium levels.

8. Herbs and spices

a. Choices

Combine basil, thyme, oregano, cumin, turmeric, and garlic powder.

b. Considerations

Sodium-free flavor enhancers. Experiment using different herbs and spices to provide variation.

9. Low-Phosphorus Fruits

a. Choices

• Apples, berries, grapes, and peaches.

b. Considerations

Choose fruits with reduced phosphorus content to manage intake.

10. Healthy oils

a. Choices

Olive, avocado, and flaxseed oils.

b. Considerations

Use to cook or drizzle on salads for heart-healthy fats.

11. Low Sodium Condiments

a. Choices

Combine mustard, vinegar, and low sodium soy sauce.

b. Considerations

Improve flavor without adding too much sodium. Check labels for concealed sodium levels.

12. Canned tomatoes and tomato products

a. Choices

Use low-sodium canned tomatoes, tomato paste, and sauce.

b. Considerations

Offers a variety of low-sodium cooking items.

13. Grain Alternatives

a. Choices

Quinoa, cauliflower rice, and spiralized veggies.

b. Considerations

Increase meal variety by substituting conventional grains.

14. Low-sodium broth:

a. Choices

Use vegetable broth or homemade broth with low salt concentration.

b. Considerations

A low-sodium soup and stew foundation.

15. Low-sugar desserts

a. Choices

Minimally sweetened frozen fruit popsicles, sorbets, and handmade sweets.

b. Considerations

Please sweet cravings without consuming too much sugar.

16. Dry Herbs for Tea

a. Choices

Tea options include nettle, chamomile, and mint.

b. Considerations

Hydrating choices with no additional potassium or phosphorus.

17. Nutritional Supplements

a. Choices

Healthcare practitioners recommend multivitamins and supplements to address specific nutrient shortages.

b. Considerations

Medical supervision is necessary while using supplements to ensure they are appropriate for particular health needs.

SELECTING LOW-POTASSIUM AND LOW-PHOSPHORUS FOODS

Individuals with Chronic renal Disease (CKD) must manage their potassium and phosphorus intake to maintain renal function and avoid problems. Choosing low-potassium and low-phosphorus foods becomes an important part of dietary management. Here is a comprehensive tutorial on how to make informed choices about essential nutrients.

Understanding potassium and phosphorus

1.Potassium

Essential for neuron and muscle cell activity, heart rhythm, and fluid balance.

Concern in CKD: Damaged kidneys may struggle to eliminate excess potassium, resulting in hyperkalemia.

2.Phosphorus

Function: Important for bone and tooth health, energy metabolism, and acid-base balance.

High phosphorus levels in CKD might cause bone and cardiac issues due to impaired renal excretion.

Choosing Low Potassium Foods

1.Fruits

Low potassium options include apples, berries (strawberries, blues, raspberries), cherries, and peaches.

Limit potassium-rich fruits such as bananas, oranges, and kiwi.

2.Vegetables

Low potassium options include bell peppers, cabbage, cauliflower, zucchini, and green beans.

Limit potassium-rich vegetables such as potatoes, tomatoes, and spinach.

3.Grains

Low-Potassium options include white rice, bread, pasta, and couscous.

Be mindful of portion control when eating whole grains, as they may contain more potassium.

4.Proteins

Low potassium options include egg whites, tofu, and skinless chicken or turkey.

Maintain a moderate protein intake and avoid high-potassium sources such as nuts, seeds, and certain legumes.

5.Dairy alternatives

Low-potassium options include rice milk, almond milk (if not phosphorus limited), and non-dairy creamer.

Consider the phosphorus content in dairy replacements.

6.Snacks

Low-Potassium options include popcorn, pretzels, and rice cakes.

Avoid snacks high in potassium, such as nuts and chocolate.

7.Beverages

Low-potassium options include water, herbal tea, and lemonade (made with low-potassium fruits).

Consider limiting potassium-rich fruit juices and sports drinks.

Choose Low-Phosphorus Foods

1.Proteins

Low-Phosphorus options include egg whites, white fish, and skinless fowl.

Limit high-phosphorus proteins, including organ meats, shellfish, and processed meats.

2.Fruits

Low-phosphorus options include apples, berries, and peaches.

Limit dry fruits and those high in phosphorus, such as oranges.

3.Vegetables

Low-phosphorus options include cabbage, green beans, and carrots.

Limit phosphorus-rich vegetables, such as potatoes and tomatoes.

4.Grains

Low-phosphorus options include white rice, bread, and pasta.

Considerations: Whole grains may contain more phosphorus; therefore moderation is important.

5.Dairy alternatives

Low-phosphorus options include unenriched rice milk and almond milk.

COOKING TECHNIQUES FOR KIDNEY-FRIENDLY MEALS

When preparing meals for people with Chronic Kidney Disease (CKD), it is critical to use cooking methods that preserve nutritional content while limiting potassium, phosphorus, and sodium intake. Kidney-friendly cooking methods are essential for generating delicious, nutritious meals that adhere to dietary restrictions. Here's a comprehensive guide to choosing and using cooking methods for kidney health.

1. Grilling

Benefits

Preserves natural tastes without excessive fats.

Suitable for lean foods such as chicken, turkey, and fish.

Considerations

Avoid using high-sodium marinades and sauces.

Consider marination with herbs, spices, and healthful oils.

2. Steaming

Benefits

Vegetables cook fast, preserving their nutrients.

Promotes heart health with minimum additional fats.

Considerations

Select low potassium veggies including cauliflower, broccoli, and green beans.

Reduce the usage of high-sodium seasoning.

3. Boiling

Benefits

Easy way to prepare grains, pasta, and vegetables.

Helps reduce potassium content in some foods.

Considerations

Use plenty of water to remove potassium.

Remove extra water to reduce potassium and sodium.

4. Baking

Benefits

Preserves tastes without overuse of oils.

Perfect for roasting veggies to enhance sweetness.

Considerations

Bake instead of fried to reduce extra fat.

Flavor can be enhanced using herbs and spices without adding salt.

5. Sautéing

Benefits

Quick and flavorful cooking method.

Uses nonstick cookware or healthy oils to reduce the need for extra fat.

Considerations

Limit sodium intake by avoiding high-sodium spices.

Add taste with healthy oils such as olive oil.

6. Slow Cooking

Benefits

Perfect for tenderizing lean meats and beans.

Perfect for adding kidney-friendly products.

Considerations

Select low-sodium broths or stocks.

Monitor phosphorus levels in slow-cooked dishes.

7. Pressure Cooking

Benefits

Reduces cooking time and preserves nutrients.

Suitable for beans, cereals, and harder cuts of meat.

Considerations

Use low-sodium broths to manage salt intake.

Adjust cooking times to reduce nutritional loss.

8. Microwaving

Benefits

Efficient for reheating and cooking veggies.

Preserves more nutrients compared to boiling.

Considerations

To keep moisture, cover food with a lid or microwave-safe wrap.

Use herbs and spices instead of high-sodium sauces.

9. Poaching

Benefits

Gentle cooking method for delicate proteins such as fish.

Preserves moisture without adding fat.

Considerations

Use low-sodium broths or water when poaching liquids.

Boost flavor with herbs, lemon, or vinegar.

10. Stir-Frying

Benefits

The quick cooking procedure maintains textures and flavors.

Use a non-stick pan to cook with less additional fat.

Considerations

Choose lean proteins and low-potassium veggies.

Be aware of salt levels in stir-fry sauces.

11. Blanching

Benefits

Quick cooking process preserves color and nutrition.

Ideal for preparing veggies before adding into meals.

Considerations

To stop cooking, briefly immerse veggies in boiling water and then immediately transfer to ice water.

Choose low-potassium vegetables to blanch.

12. Griddle or Pan-Sear

Benefits

Produces a caramelized exterior without excessive fats.

Suitable for lean meats and certain vegetables.

Considerations

Choose lean proteins and low potassium veggies.

Minimize oil and sodium content in seasonings.

CHAPTER 1

Breakfast recipes

1.Quinoa Breakfast Bowl with Berries and Almonds

Health Benefits

- Quinoa provides a complete protein source with essential amino acids.

- Berries offer antioxidants and are low in potassium.

- Almonds contribute healthy fats and a crunch to the dish.

Ingredients

- 1 cup cooked quinoa

- Mixed berries (strawberries, blueberries, raspberries) of 1/2 cup

- 2 tablespoons sliced almonds

- 1 tablespoon maple syrup (optional)

Mode of Preparation

1. Cook quinoa according to package instructions.

2. In a bowl, combine cooked quinoa, mixed berries, and sliced almonds.

3. Drizzle with maple syrup if desired.

4. Gently toss and serve.

Nutritional Information

- Protein: 10g

- Fiber: 6g

- Potassium: 150mg

- Phosphorus: 120mg

Serving Size: 1 bowl

Cooking Time: 15 minutes

Preparation Time: 5 minutes

2.Chia Seed Pudding with Mango and Coconut

Health Benefits

- Chia seeds are rich in omega-3 fatty acids and low in potassium.

- Mango provides vitamins and antioxidants.

- Coconut adds flavor without excess phosphorus.

Ingredients

- 3 tablespoons chia seeds

- 1 cup unsweetened almond milk

- 1/2 cup diced ripe mango

- 1 tablespoon shredded coconut

Mode of Preparation

1. Chia seeds and almond milk should be mixed in a bowl.

2. It should be Refrigerated for at least 4 hours or overnight.

3. Once the chia pudding has set, layer it with diced mango and shredded coconut.

4. Repeat the layers and serve.

Nutritional Information

- Protein: 6g

- Fiber: 10g

- Potassium: 180mg

- Phosphorus: 80mg

Serving Size: 1 serving

Cooking Time: 4 hours (for chia pudding to set)

Preparation Time: 10 minutes

3.Sweet Potato and Spinach Breakfast Hash

Health Benefits

- Sweet potatoes are a good source of vitamins and low in potassium.

- Spinach provides iron and folate.

- Chickpeas add plant-based protein.

Ingredients

- 1 medium sweet potato, diced

- 1 cup fresh spinach

- Canned chickpeas, drained and rinsed of 1/2 cup

- 1 tablespoon olive oil

- Salt and pepper to taste

Mode of Preparation

1. Olive oil should be heated in a skillet over medium heat.

2. Add diced sweet potatoes and cook until they start to brown.

3. Add chickpeas and spinach, cooking until spinach wilts.

4. Add salt and pepper to taste.

Nutritional Information

- Protein: 8g

- Fiber: 7g

- Potassium: 200mg

- Phosphorus: 90mg

Serving Size: 1 serving

Cooking Time: 20 minutes

Preparation Time: 10 minutes

4.Oatmeal with Apple and Cinnamon

Health Benefits

- Oats provide soluble fiber and are kidney-friendly.

- Apples offer dietary fiber and antioxidants.

- Cinnamon adds flavor without additional nutrients.

Ingredients

- 1/2 cup rolled oats

- 1 medium apple, diced

- 1/2 teaspoon ground cinnamon

- 1 tablespoon almond butter

Mode of Preparation

1. Cook oats according to package instructions.

2. Stir in diced apples and ground cinnamon.

3. Top with a dollop of almond butter.

Nutritional Information

- Protein: 7g

- Fiber: 5g

- Potassium: 180mg

- Phosphorus: 80mg

Serving Size: 1 serving

Cooking Time: 10 minutes

Preparation Time: 5 minutes

5.Avocado and Tomato Toast

Health Benefits

- Avocado provides healthy fats and is low in potassium.

- Tomatoes offer vitamins and antioxidants.

- Whole grain bread contributes fiber.

Ingredients

- 1 slice whole grain bread

- 1/2 ripe avocado, mashed

- 1 medium tomato, sliced

- Salt and pepper to taste

- Fresh basil leaves for garnish (optional)

Mode of Preparation

1. Whole grain bread should be toasted to your liking.

2. Spread mashed avocado on the toast.

3. Top with sliced tomatoes.

4. Season with salt and pepper, and garnish with fresh basil if desired.

Nutritional Information

- Protein: 5g

- Fiber: 8g

- Potassium: 220mg

- Phosphorus: 100mg

Serving Size: 1 serving

Cooking Time: 5 minutes

Preparation Time: 5 minutes

6: Lentil and Vegetable Scramble

Health Benefits

- Lentils are a great plant-based protein source low in potassium.

- Mixed vegetables add vitamins and fiber.

- Turmeric provides anti-inflammatory properties.

Ingredients

- Cooked green or brown lentils of 1/2 cup.

- 1/2 cup mixed vegetables (bell peppers, zucchini, spinach)

- 1/4 teaspoon turmeric powder

- 1 tablespoon olive oil

- Salt and pepper to taste

Mode of Preparation

1. Olive oil should be heated in a pan over medium heat.

2. Mixed vegetables should be added and sauté until tender.

3. Stir in cooked lentils and turmeric powder.

4. Add salt and pepper to taste.

Nutritional Information

- Protein: 9g

- Fiber: 8g

- Potassium: 230mg

- Phosphorus: 120mg

Serving Size: 1 serving

Cooking Time: 15 minutes

Preparation Time: 10 minutes

7: Banana and Almond Butter Smoothie Bowl

Health Benefits

- Bananas are low in potassium and provide natural sweetness.

- Almond butter gives us healthy fats and protein.

- Spinach contributes iron without excess phosphorus.

Ingredients

- 1 ripe banana

- 1 tablespoon almond butter

- 1/2 cup fresh spinach

- 1/2 cup unsweetened almond milk

- Toppings: sliced strawberries, chia seeds

Mode of Preparation

1. Blend banana, almond butter, spinach, and almond milk until smooth.

2. Pour into a bowl and top with sliced strawberries and chia seeds.

Nutritional Information

- Protein: 6g

- Fiber: 7g

- Potassium: 220mg

- Phosphorus: 100mg

Serving Size: 1 bowl

Cooking Time: 5 minutes

Preparation Time: 5 minutes

8: Millet Porridge with Mixed Berries

Health Benefits

- Millet is a low-potassium grain rich in fiber.

- Mixed berries offer antioxidants and vitamins.

- Coconut milk adds creaminess without dairy.

Ingredients

- 1/2 cup millet

- 1 1/2 cups water

- Mixed berries (strawberries, blueberries, raspberries) of 1/2 cup

- 2 tablespoons coconut milk

- 1 tablespoon maple syrup (optional)

Mode of Preparation

1. Rinse millet under cold water.

2. Combine millet and water in a pot.

3. It should be brought to a boil, then simmer until water is absorbed.

4. Stir in mixed berries, coconut milk, and maple syrup if desired.

Nutritional Information

- Protein: 7g

- Fiber: 5g

- Potassium: 160mg

- Phosphorus: 80mg

Serving Size: 1 serving

Cooking Time: 25 minutes

Preparation Time: 10 minutes

9: Cauliflower and Kale Breakfast Wrap

Health Benefits

- Cauliflower is low in potassium and provides a grain-free alternative.

- Kale adds vitamins and minerals.

- Hummus contributes plant-based protein.

Ingredients

- 1 cauliflower tortilla

- 1 cup chopped kale

- 2 tablespoons hummus

- 1/4 cup cherry tomatoes, halved

- Salt and pepper to taste

Mode of Preparation

1. In a pan, sauté kale until wilted.

2. Spread hummus on the cauliflower tortilla.

3. Add sautéed kale and halved cherry tomatoes.

4. Season with salt and pepper, then roll into a wrap.

Nutritional Information

- Protein: 8g

- Fiber: 6g

- Potassium: 190mg

- Phosphorus: 90mg

Serving Size: 1 wrap

Cooking Time: 10 minutes

Preparation Time: 5 minutes

10: Mango and Avocado Smoothie

Health Benefits

- Mango provides natural sweetness and vitamins.

- Avocado adds healthy fats and creaminess.

- Almond milk offers a dairy-free base.

Ingredients

- 1 ripe mango, peeled and diced

- 1/2 avocado, peeled and pitted

- 1 cup unsweetened almond milk

- 1 tablespoon chia seeds

- Ice cubes (optional)

Mode of Preparation

1. Blend mango, avocado, almond milk, and chia seeds until smooth.

2. Add ice cubes if a colder consistency is desired.

Nutritional Information

- Protein: 5g

- Fiber: 9g

- Potassium: 210mg

- Phosphorus: 110mg

Serving Size: 1 glass

Cooking Time: 5 minutes

Preparation Time: 5 minutes

11: Rice Paper Rolls with Tofu and Vegetables

Health Benefits

- Rice paper provides a low-potassium wrapper.

- Tofu adds plant-based protein without excessive phosphorus.

- Colorful vegetables offer vitamins and fiber.

Ingredients

- 4 rice paper sheets

- 1/2 cup firm tofu, sliced

- 1/2 cup cucumber, julienned

- 1/2 cup carrot, julienned

- 1/4 cup fresh mint leaves

- 2 tablespoons hoisin sauce (low-sodium)

Mode of Preparation

1. Soften rice paper sheets in warm water according to package instructions.

2. Lay each sheet flat and fill with tofu, cucumber, carrot, and mint leaves.

3. Roll tightly, tucking in the sides, and serve with hoisin sauce.

Nutritional Information

- Protein: 8g

- Fiber: 3g

- Potassium: 190mg

- Phosphorus: 100mg

Serving Size: 1 serving (2 rolls)

Cooking Time: 15 minutes

Preparation Time: 20 minutes

12: Blueberry and Walnut Overnight Oats

Health Benefits

- Oats offer soluble fiber for digestive health.

- Blueberries provide antioxidants and are low in potassium.

- Walnuts contribute omega-3 fatty acids.

Ingredients

- 1/2 cup rolled oats

- 1/2 cup unsweetened almond milk

- 1/4 cup fresh blueberries

- 1 tablespoon chopped walnuts

- 1 teaspoon maple syrup (optional)

Mode of Preparation

1. Mix rolled oats and almond milk in a jar or container.

2. Add blueberries and chopped walnuts.

3. Seal and refrigerate overnight.

4. Drizzle with maple syrup if desired before serving.

Nutritional Information

- Protein: 6g

- Fiber: 5g

- Potassium: 170mg

- Phosphorus: 90mg

Serving Size: 1 serving

Cooking Time: Overnight (refrigeration)

Preparation Time: 5 minutes

13: Cinnamon-Roasted Butternut Squash Bowl

Health Benefits

- Butternut squash is low in potassium and high in vitamins.

- Cinnamon adds flavor without additional nutrients.

- Quinoa provides protein and fiber.

Ingredients

- 1 cup cubed butternut squash

- 1 teaspoon olive oil

- 1/2 teaspoon ground cinnamon

- 1/2 cup cooked quinoa

- 1 tablespoon pumpkin seeds

- Drizzle of balsamic glaze (optional)

Mode of Preparation

1. Toss cubed butternut squash in olive oil and cinnamon.

2. Roast in the oven until tender.

3. Serve over cooked quinoa, topped with pumpkin seeds.

4. Drizzle with balsamic glaze if desired.

Nutritional Information

- Protein: 7g

- Fiber: 6g

- Potassium: 210mg

- Phosphorus: 100mg

Serving Size: 1 serving

Cooking Time: 30 minutes

Preparation Time: 15 minutes

14: Chickpea and Vegetable Stir-Fry

Health Benefits

- Chickpeas offer plant-based protein and fiber.

- Colorful vegetables provide vitamins and minerals.

- Stir-frying retains nutrients with minimal added fats.

Ingredients

- 1 cup cooked chickpeas

- Mixed vegetables (broccoli, bell peppers, snap peas) of 1 cup

- 1 tablespoon soy sauce (low-sodium)

- 1 tablespoon sesame oil

- 1/2 teaspoon ginger, minced

Mode of Preparation

1. In a wok or pan, heat sesame oil over medium heat.

2. Add mixed vegetables and stir-fry until crisp-tender.

3. Add cooked chickpeas and minced ginger.

4. Pour in low-sodium soy sauce and toss until heated through.

Nutritional Information

- Protein: 10g

- Fiber: 8g

- Potassium: 240mg

- Phosphorus: 110mg

Serving Size: 1 serving

Cooking Time: 15 minutes

Preparation Time: 10 minutes

15: Pumpkin and Cacao Smoothie

Health Benefits

- Pumpkin is low in potassium and high in fiber.

- Cacao adds antioxidants and a chocolatey flavor.

- Flaxseeds contribute omega-3 fatty acids.

Ingredients

- 1/2 cup canned pumpkin puree

- 1 tablespoon cacao powder

- 1 tablespoon flaxseeds

- 1 banana, frozen

- 1 cup unsweetened coconut milk

Mode of Preparation

1. Blend pumpkin puree, cacao powder, flaxseeds, frozen banana, and coconut milk until smooth.

2. Adjust consistency with more coconut milk if needed.

Nutritional Information

- Protein: 5g

- Fiber: 8g

- Potassium: 230mg

- Phosphorus: 120mg

Serving Size: 1 glass

Cooking Time: 5 minutes

Preparation Time: 5 minutes

16: Cranberry and Walnut Quinoa Porridge

Health Benefits

- Quinoa provides protein and essential amino acids.

- Cranberries offer antioxidants and a burst of tartness.

- Walnuts contribute omega-3 fatty acids.

Ingredients

- 1/2 cup cooked quinoa

- 2 tablespoons dried cranberries

- 1 tablespoon chopped walnuts

- 1/2 teaspoon ground cinnamon

- 1 cup almond milk (unsweetened)

Mode of Preparation

1. Mix cooked quinoa, dried cranberries, chopped walnuts, and ground cinnamon in a bowl.

2. Heat almond milk and pour over the quinoa mixture.

3. Stir well and let it sit for a few minutes before serving.

Nutritional Information

- Protein: 8g

- Fiber: 5g

- Potassium: 190mg

- Phosphorus: 100mg

Serving Size: 1 serving

Cooking Time: 10 minutes

Preparation Time: 5 minutes

17: Mushroom and Spinach Breakfast Wrap

Health Benefits

- Mushrooms provide a meaty texture without high potassium.

- Spinach adds vitamins and minerals.

- Hummus contributes plant-based protein.

Ingredients

- 1 whole wheat tortilla

- 1/2 cup sliced mushrooms

- 1 cup fresh spinach

- 2 tablespoons hummus

- Salt and pepper to taste

Mode of Preparation

1. In a pan, sauté sliced mushrooms until golden brown.

2. Add fresh spinach and cook until wilted.

3. Spread hummus on the whole wheat tortilla.

4. Add the mushroom and spinach mixture. Season with salt and pepper.

5. Roll into a wrap and serve.

Nutritional Information

- Protein: 9g

- Fiber: 6g

- Potassium: 200mg

- Phosphorus: 90mg

Serving Size: 1 wrap

Cooking Time: 10 minutes

Preparation Time: 5 minutes

18: Orange and Almond Breakfast Quinoa

Health Benefits

- Quinoa provides protein and essential amino acids.

- Oranges offer vitamin C and natural sweetness.

- Almonds contribute healthy fats.

Ingredients

- 1/2 cup cooked quinoa

- 1 orange, segmented

- 1 tablespoon sliced almonds

- 1 teaspoon honey (optional)

- 1/4 teaspoon vanilla extract

Mode of Preparation

1. Mix cooked quinoa, orange segments, sliced almonds, honey (if using), and vanilla extract in a bowl.

2. Stir well and serve.

Nutritional Information

- Protein: 7g

- Fiber: 6g

- Potassium: 160mg

- Phosphorus: 80mg

Serving Size: 1 serving

Cooking Time: 15 minutes

Preparation Time: 5 minutes

19: Sweet Potato and Black Bean Breakfast Burrito

Health Benefits

- Sweet potatoes are rich in vitamins and low in potassium.

- A good source of plant-based protein and fiber is Black beans

- Whole grain tortillas add dietary fiber.

Ingredients

- 1 medium sweet potato, cubed and roasted

- 1/2 cup black beans, cooked

- 1 whole grain tortilla

- 2 tablespoons salsa (low-sodium)

- 1 tablespoon guacamole

Mode of Preparation

1. Roast cubed sweet potatoes until tender.

2. In a whole grain tortilla, layer roasted sweet potatoes and black beans.

3. Top with salsa and guacamole.

4. Roll into a burrito and serve.

Nutritional Information

- Protein: 8g

- Fiber: 7g

- Potassium: 230mg

- Phosphorus: 120mg

Serving Size: 1 burrito

Cooking Time: 30 minutes

Preparation Time: 15 minutes

CHAPTER 2

Lunch Recipes

1. Quinoa and Vegetable Buddha Bowl

Health Benefits

- Rich in plant-based proteins, essential for kidney health.

- Digestion and regulating of blood sugar levels is aided by high fiber content.

- Loaded with antioxidants from colorful vegetables, combating inflammation.

Ingredients

- 1 cup quinoa, rinsed

- 2 cups broccoli florets

- 1 cup cherry tomatoes, halved

- 1 cup shredded carrots

- 1 cup cucumber, diced

- 1 cup cooked chickpeas

- 2 tablespoons olive oil

- 1 tablespoon balsamic vinegar

- Salt and pepper to taste

Mode of Preparation

1. Cook quinoa according to package instructions.

2. Steam broccoli until tender-crisp.

3. In a large bowl, combine quinoa, broccoli, cherry tomatoes, carrots, cucumber, and chickpeas.

4. Whisk together olive oil, balsamic vinegar, salt, and pepper. Drizzle over the bowl and toss gently.

5. Serve immediately or refrigerate for later.

Nutritional Information

- Calories: 400

- Protein: 15g

- Fiber: 10g

- Potassium: 450mg

- Phosphorus: 150mg

Serving Size: 4

Cooking Time: 20 minutes

Preparation Time: 15 minutes

2. Mushroom and Spinach Stuffed Bell Peppers

Health Benefits

- Low in potassium and phosphorus, suitable for CKD patients.

- Spinach provides iron without contributing to excessive phosphorus intake.

- Mushrooms offer plant-based protein and a rich umami flavor.

Ingredients

- Halved 4 bell pepper after the seed has been removed

- 2 cups baby spinach, chopped

- 1 cup mushrooms, finely chopped

- 1 cup cooked quinoa

- 1 clove garlic, minced

- 1 teaspoon olive oil

- 1 teaspoon Italian seasoning

- Salt and pepper to taste

Mode of Preparation

1. Preheat oven to 375°F (190°C).

2. In a pan, sauté garlic in olive oil until fragrant.

3. Add mushrooms and spinach, cooking until wilted.

4. In a bowl, combine cooked quinoa, sautéed vegetables, Italian seasoning, salt, and pepper.

5. Stuff bell peppers with the mixture and place them in a baking dish.

6. Bake for 25-30 minutes until peppers are tender.

Nutritional Information

- Calories: 180

- Protein: 8g

- Fiber: 6g

- Potassium: 250mg

- Phosphorus: 120mg

Serving Size: 4

Cooking Time: 30 minutes

Preparation Time: 20 minutes

3. Lentil and Vegetable Stir-Fry

Health Benefits

- Lentils provide a low-phosphorus protein source.

- Vegetables provides us with vitamins and minerals.

- Stir-frying retains nutrients while adding flavor without excess sodium.

Ingredients

- 1 cup dried green lentils, cooked

- 2 cups broccoli florets

- 1 bell pepper, sliced

- 1 cup snap peas, trimmed

- 1 carrot, julienned

- 2 tablespoons low-sodium soy sauce

- 1 tablespoon sesame oil

- 1 teaspoon ginger, minced

- 1 clove garlic, minced

- 1 tablespoon sesame seeds (for garnish)

Mode of Preparation

1. Cook lentils according to package instructions.

2. In a wok or large skillet, heat sesame oil over medium-high heat.

3. Add ginger and garlic, stir-frying for 30 seconds.

4. Add broccoli, bell pepper, snap peas, and carrot, stir-frying until vegetables are crisp-tender.

5. Add cooked lentils and soy sauce, tossing to combine.

6. Garnish with sesame seeds and serve over brown rice.

Nutritional Information

- Calories: 250

- Protein: 15g

- Fiber: 8g

- Potassium: 300mg

- Phosphorus: 150mg

Serving Size: 4

Cooking Time: 15 minutes

Preparation Time: 20 minutes

4. Sweet Potato and Chickpea Curry

Health Benefits

- Sweet potatoes offer a potassium-friendly alternative to regular potatoes.

- Chickpeas provide plant-based protein and fiber.

- Turmeric and ginger in the curry offer anti-inflammatory properties.

Ingredients

- Sweet potatoes (2), peeled and diced

- 1 can (15 oz) chickpeas, drained and rinsed

- 1 onion, finely chopped

- 2 cloves garlic, minced

- 1 can (14 oz) diced tomatoes

- 1 can (14 oz) coconut milk

- 2 tablespoons curry powder

- 1 teaspoon turmeric

- 1 teaspoon ginger, grated

- Salt and pepper to taste

- Fresh cilantro (for garnish)

Mode of Preparation

1. In a large pot, sauté onion and garlic until softened.

2. Add sweet potatoes, chickpeas, diced tomatoes, coconut milk, curry powder, turmeric, ginger, salt, and pepper.

3. Bring to a boil, then reduce heat and simmer until sweet potatoes are tender.

4. Garnish with fresh cilantro and serve over quinoa or brown rice.

Nutritional Information

- Calories: 300

- Protein: 10g

- Fiber: 9g

- Potassium: 400mg

- Phosphorus: 180mg

Serving Size: 4

Cooking Time: 40 minutes

Preparation Time: 25 minutes

5. Cauliflower and Chickpea Salad with Lemon Tahini Dressing

Health Benefits

- Cauliflower is a low-potassium and low-phosphorus cruciferous vegetable.

- Chickpeas contribute plant-based protein and fiber.

- Lemon tahini dressing adds a burst of flavor without excess sodium.

Ingredients

- 1 medium cauliflower, cut into florets

- 1 can (15 oz) chickpeas, drained and rinsed

- 1 cucumber, diced

- 1 cup cherry tomatoes, halved

- 1/2 red onion, thinly sliced

- 1/4 cup fresh parsley, chopped

- 1/4 cup tahini

- Juice of 1 lemon

- 2 tablespoons olive oil

- Salt and pepper to taste

Mode of Preparation

1. Steam cauliflower until tender-crisp.

2. In a large bowl, combine cauliflower, chickpeas, cucumber, cherry tomatoes, red onion, and parsley.

3. In a small bowl, whisk together tahini, lemon juice, olive oil, salt, and pepper.

4. Dressing should be drizzled over the salad and toss gently to combine.

5. It should be Refrigerated for at least 30 minutes before serving.

Nutritional Information

- Calories: 280

- Protein: 12g

- Fiber: 8g

- Potassium: 350mg

- Phosphorus: 160mg

Serving Size: 4

Cooking Time: 15 minutes

Preparation Time: 20 minutes

6. Mediterranean Chickpea Salad

Health Benefits

- Chickpeas provide plant-based protein without excess phosphorus.

- Colorful bell peppers and cherry tomatoes offer antioxidants.

- Olive oil contributes heart-healthy monounsaturated fats.

Ingredients

- Chickpeas of 2 cans (15 oz each), drained and rinsed

- 1 cucumber, diced

- 1 cup cherry tomatoes, halved

- 1 red bell pepper, diced

- 1 yellow bell pepper, diced

- 1/2 red onion, finely chopped

- 1/4 cup Kalamata olives, sliced

- 1/4 cup fresh parsley, chopped

- 2 tablespoons extra-virgin olive oil

- Juice of 1 lemon

- 1 teaspoon dried oregano

- Salt and pepper to taste

Mode of Preparation

1. In a large bowl, combine chickpeas, cucumber, cherry tomatoes, bell peppers, red onion, olives, and parsley.

2. Whisk together olive oil, lemon juice, dried oregano, salt, and pepper in a bowl.

3. The dressing should be poured over the salad and toss gently.

4. Leave in the refrigerator for at least 30 minutes before serving.

Nutritional Information

- Calories: 300

- Protein: 12g

- Fiber: 10g

- Potassium: 350mg

- Phosphorus: 180mg

Serving Size: 4

Cooking Time: 15 minutes

Preparation Time: 20 minutes

7. Spaghetti Squash Primavera

Health Benefits

- Spaghetti squash is a low-potassium alternative to traditional pasta.

- Assorted vegetables provide a range of vitamins and minerals.

- Olive oil provide us with healthy fats, beneficial for heart health.

Ingredients

- 1 medium spaghetti squash

- 2 tablespoons olive oil

- 1 onion, thinly sliced

- 2 cloves garlic, minced

- 1 bell pepper, thinly sliced

- 1 zucchini, julienned

- 1 cup cherry tomatoes, halved

- 1 cup baby spinach

- 1/4 cup fresh basil, chopped

- Salt and pepper to taste

- Vegan Parmesan (optional, for garnish)

Mode of Preparation

1. Preheat the oven to 375°F (190°C).

2. Cut the spaghetti squash in half lengthwise, remove seeds, and place it on a baking sheet.

3. Roast for 40-45 minutes or until the squash is tender.

4. Olive oil should be heated in a large skillet over medium heat.

5. Onion and garlic should be added, sautéing until softened.

6. Add bell pepper, zucchini, cherry tomatoes, and spinach, cooking until vegetables are tender.

7. Scrape the spaghetti squash flesh with a fork to create "noodles" and add them to the skillet.

8. Toss everything together, add basil, salt, and pepper. Garnish with vegan Parmesan if desired.

Nutritional Information

- Calories: 250

- Protein: 6g

- Fiber: 8g

- Potassium: 300mg

- Phosphorus: 120mg

Serving Size: 4

Cooking Time: 1 hour

Preparation Time: 20 minutes

8. Black Bean and Corn Stuffed Peppers

Health Benefits

- Black beans provide plant-based protein with low phosphorus content.

- Corn adds natural sweetness and fiber to the dish.

- Bell peppers offer vitamin C and A, supporting immune health.

Ingredients

- Halved 4 bell pepper after the seed has been removed

- 2 cups cooked black beans

- Corn kernels (fresh or frozen) of 1 cup

- 1 cup cherry tomatoes, diced

- 1/2 red onion, finely chopped

- 1 jalapeño, minced (optional for heat)

- 1 teaspoon ground cumin

- 1 teaspoon chili powder

- Salt and pepper to taste

- Fresh cilantro (for garnish)

Mode of Preparation

1. Preheat the oven to 375°F (190°C).

2. In a bowl, combine black beans, corn, cherry tomatoes, red onion, jalapeño, cumin, chili powder, salt, and pepper.

3. Each bell pepper half should be stuff with the mixture and place them in a baking dish.

4. Bake for 25-30 minutes or until the peppers are tender.

5. Garnish with fresh cilantro before serving.

Nutritional Information

- Calories: 280

- Protein: 12g

- Fiber: 9g

- Potassium: 350mg

- Phosphorus: 160mg

Serving Size: 4

Cooking Time: 30 minutes

Preparation Time: 20 minute

9. Lentil and Vegetable Soup
Health Benefits

- Lentils provide a low-phosphorus, high-fiber protein source.

- Assorted vegetables offer vitamins, minerals, and antioxidants.

- Low sodium content supports kidney health.

Ingredients

- 1 cup dry green or brown lentils, rinsed

- 1 onion, diced

- 2 carrots, diced

- 2 celery stalks, diced

- 2 cloves garlic, minced

- 1 can (14 oz) diced tomatoes (low-sodium)

- 6 cups vegetable broth (low-sodium)

- 1 teaspoon dried thyme

- 1 teaspoon dried rosemary

- Salt and pepper to taste

- 2 cups spinach, chopped (optional)

Mode of Preparation

1. In a large pot, sauté onion, carrots, celery, and garlic until softened.

2. Add lentils, diced tomatoes, vegetable broth, thyme, rosemary, salt, and pepper.

3. Bring to a boil, then reduce heat and simmer for 25-30 minutes or until lentils are tender.

4. Chopped spinach should be added and cook until wilted.

5. Adjust seasoning as needed and serve.

Nutritional Information

- Calories: 150

- Protein: 9g

- Fiber: 8g

- Potassium: 250mg

- Phosphorus: 120mg

Serving Size: 6

Cooking Time: 40 minutes

Preparation Time: 15 minutes

10. Roasted Vegetable Quinoa Bowl

Health Benefits

- Quinoa provides a complete protein source with low phosphorus.

- Roasted vegetables offer a variety of vitamins and minerals.

- Olive oil adds heart-healthy monounsaturated fats.

Ingredients

- 1 cup quinoa, rinsed

- 1 sweet potato, diced

- 1 zucchini, sliced

- 1 bell pepper, diced

- 1 red onion, sliced

- 2 tablespoons olive oil

- 1 teaspoon dried thyme

- 1 teaspoon paprika

- Salt and pepper to taste

- 1/4 cup fresh parsley, chopped

Mode of Preparation

1. Preheat the oven to 400°F (200°C).

2. Toss sweet potato, zucchini, bell pepper, and red onion with olive oil, thyme, paprika, salt, and pepper.

3. Roast the vegetables for 25-30 minutes or until golden and tender.

4. Cook quinoa according to package instructions.

5. Serve quinoa topped with roasted vegetables and garnish with fresh parsley.

Nutritional Information

- Calories: 280

- Protein: 8g

- Fiber: 6g

- Potassium: 300mg

- Phosphorus: 150mg

Serving Size: 4

Cooking Time: 30 minutes

Preparation Time: 20 minutes

11. Chickpea and Avocado Wrap

Health Benefits

- Chickpeas offer plant-based protein and fiber.

- Avocado provides healthy monounsaturated fats.

- Whole-grain wraps offer additional fiber and nutrients.

Ingredients

- 1 can (15 oz) chickpeas, drained and rinsed

- 1 avocado, mashed

- 1/4 cup red onion, finely chopped

- 1/4 cup fresh cilantro, chopped

- Juice of 1 lime

- Salt and pepper to taste

- 4 whole-grain wraps

- 2 cups mixed greens

- 1 tomato, sliced

Mode of Preparation

1. In a bowl, combine chickpeas, mashed avocado, red onion, cilantro, lime juice, salt, and pepper.

2. Lay out whole-grain wraps and divide the chickpea mixture evenly among them.

3. Top each wrap with mixed greens and tomato slices.

4. Fold the wraps and secure with toothpicks if needed.

5. Serve immediately or wrap in parchment paper for later.

Nutritional Information

- Calories: 320

- Protein: 10g

- Fiber: 8g

- Potassium: 400mg

- Phosphorus: 180mg

Serving Size: 4

Cooking Time: 15 minutes

Preparation Time: 10 minutes

12. Spinach and Artichoke Quiche

Health Benefits

- Spinach is a low-potassium leafy green rich in iron and vitamins.

- Artichokes contribute dietary fiber and antioxidants.

- Tofu provides a plant-based protein source.

Ingredients

- 1 pre-made whole wheat pie crust

- 1 cup fresh spinach, chopped

- Artichoke hearts of 1 can (14 oz), drained and chopped

- Firm tofu of 1 block (14 oz), crumbled

- 1/2 cup nutritional yeast

- 1/2 cup unsweetened almond milk

- 2 tablespoons olive oil

- 2 cloves garlic, minced

- 1 teaspoon dried thyme

- Salt and pepper to taste

Mode of Preparation

1. Preheat the oven to 375°F (190°C).

2. In a skillet, sauté garlic in olive oil until fragrant. Add spinach and cook until wilted.

3. In a blender, combine crumbled tofu, nutritional yeast, almond milk, thyme, salt, and pepper. Blend until smooth.

4. Mix the tofu mixture with sautéed spinach and chopped artichokes.

5. Pour the mixture into the pie crust and bake for 30-35 minutes or until set.

6. Make it cool down before slicing and serving.

Nutritional Information

- Calories: 220

- Protein: 12g

- Fiber: 4g

- Potassium: 300mg

- Phosphorus: 150mg

Serving Size: 8

Cooking Time: 35 minutes

Preparation Time: 20 minutes

13. Mediterranean Chickpea and Quinoa Salad

Health Benefits

- Chickpeas and quinoa provide a protein-packed base.

- Vegetables provides vitamins and antioxidants.

- Olive oil and lemon dressing adds healthy fats and flavor.

Ingredients

- 1 cup cooked quinoa

- 1 can (15 oz) chickpeas, drained and rinsed

- 1 cucumber, diced

- 1 cup cherry tomatoes, halved

- 1 red bell pepper, diced

- 1/2 red onion, finely chopped

- 1/4 cup Kalamata olives, sliced

- 1/4 cup fresh parsley, chopped

- 2 tablespoons extra-virgin olive oil

- Juice of 1 lemon

- 1 teaspoon dried oregano

- Salt and pepper to taste

Mode of Preparation

1. In a large bowl, combine cooked quinoa, chickpeas, cucumber, cherry tomatoes, bell pepper, red onion, olives, and parsley.

2. Whisk together olive oil, lemon juice, dried oregano, salt, and pepper in a small bowl.

3. Dressing should be poured over the salad and toss gently.

4. Leave in the refrigerator for at least 30 minutes before serving.

Nutritional Information

- Calories: 300

- Protein: 12g

- Fiber: 10g

- Potassium: 350mg

- Phosphorus: 180mg

Serving Size: 4

Cooking Time: 20 minutes

Preparation Time: 15 minutes

14. Sweet Potato and Black Bean Quesadillas

Health Benefits

- Sweet potatoes provide a potassium-friendly alternative to regular potatoes.

- Black beans provides with plant-based protein and fiber

- Whole-grain tortillas add additional fiber and nutrients.

Ingredients

- Sweet potatoes (2), peeled and diced

- Black beans of 1 can (15 oz) , drained and rinsed

- 1 teaspoon ground cumin

- 1 teaspoon chili powder

- Salt and pepper to taste

- 4 whole-grain tortillas

- 1 cup vegan cheese, shredded

- 1 avocado, sliced

- Fresh cilantro (for garnish)

Mode of Preparation

1. Steam or roast sweet potatoes until tender.

2. In a bowl, mash black beans and combine with cooked sweet potatoes, cumin, chili powder, salt, and pepper.

3. Lay out tortillas and divide the sweet potato and black bean mixture evenly among them.

4. Sprinkle vegan cheese on top and fold the tortillas in half.

5. Cook quesadillas on a skillet over medium heat until cheese is melted and tortillas are crispy.

6. Top with sliced avocado and fresh cilantro before serving.

Nutritional Information

- Calories: 350

- Protein: 12g

- Fiber: 8g

- Potassium: 400mg

- Phosphorus: 180mg

Serving Size: 4

Cooking Time: 25 minutes

Preparation Time: 20 minutes

15. Broccoli and Red Lentil Soup

Health Benefits

- Red lentils are a low-phosphorus protein source.

- Broccoli adds vitamins, minerals, and antioxidants.

- Low-sodium vegetable broth supports kidney health.

Ingredients

- 1 cup red lentils, rinsed

- 1 onion, diced

- 2 carrots, diced

- 2 celery stalks, diced

- 3 cups broccoli florets

- 2 cloves garlic, minced

- 6 cups low-sodium vegetable broth

- 1 teaspoon cumin

- 1 teaspoon turmeric

- Salt and pepper to taste

- Fresh parsley (for garnish)

Mode of Preparation

1. In a large pot, sauté onion, carrots, celery, and garlic until softened.

2. Add red lentils, broccoli, vegetable broth, cumin, turmeric, salt, and pepper.

3. Bring to a boil, then reduce heat and simmer for 20-25 minutes or until lentils are tender.

4. Blend the soup until smooth using an immersion blender or traditional blender.

5. Garnish with fresh parsley and serve.

Nutritional Information

-   Calories: 180

-   Protein: 10g

-   Fiber: 8g

-   Potassium: 250mg

-   Phosphorus: 120mg

Serving Size: 6

Cooking Time: 30 minutes

Preparation Time: 15 minutes

16. Portobello Mushroom and Quinoa Stuffed Peppers

Health Benefits

- Quinoa provides a complete protein source.

- Portobello mushrooms offer a meaty texture without excess phosphorus.

- Bell peppers provide vitamins and antioxidants.

Ingredients

- Halved 4 bell pepper after the seed has been removed

- 1 cup cooked quinoa

- 2 portobello mushrooms, chopped

- 1 onion, finely chopped

- 2 cloves garlic, minced

- 1 can (14 oz) diced tomatoes (low-sodium)

- 1 teaspoon dried thyme

- 1 teaspoon smoked paprika

- Salt and pepper to taste

- Vegan cheese (optional, for topping)

Mode of Preparation

1. Preheat the oven to 375°F (190°C).

2. In a skillet, sauté onion and garlic until softened. Add portobello mushrooms and cook until tender.

3. Stir in cooked quinoa, diced tomatoes, thyme, smoked paprika, salt, and pepper.

4. Stuff each bell pepper half with the mixture and place them in a baking dish.

5. Optional: Top with vegan cheese.

6. It should be baked for 25-30 minutes or until the peppers are tender.

Nutritional Information

- Calories: 250

- Protein: 10g

- Fiber: 6g

- Potassium: 300mg

- Phosphorus: 150mg

Serving Size: 4

Cooking Time: 30 minutes

Preparation Time: 20 minutes

17. Mediterranean Quinoa Salad with Lemon-Tahini Dressing

Health Benefits

- Quinoa provides a nutrient-dense, low-phosphorus base.

- Mediterranean vegetables offer a variety of vitamins and minerals.

- Lemon-tahini dressing adds flavor without excess sodium.

Ingredients

- 1 cup cooked quinoa

- 1 cucumber, diced

- 1 cup cherry tomatoes, halved

- 1 bell pepper, diced

- 1/2 red onion, finely chopped

- 1/4 cup Kalamata olives, sliced

- 1/4 cup fresh parsley, chopped

- 2 tablespoons tahini

- Juice of 1 lemon

- 2 tablespoons olive oil

- 1 teaspoon dried oregano

- Salt and pepper to taste

Mode of Preparation

1. In a large bowl, combine cooked quinoa, cucumber, cherry tomatoes, bell pepper, red onion, olives, and parsley.

2. In a small bowl, whisk together tahini, lemon juice, olive oil, dried oregano, salt, and pepper.

3. Dressing should be poured over the salad and toss gently.

4. It should be Refrigerated for at least 30 minutes before serving.

Nutritional Information

- Calories: 300

- Protein: 10g

- Fiber: 8g

- Potassium: 350mg

- Phosphorus: 160mg

Serving Size: 4

Cooking Time: 20 minutes

Preparation Time: 15 minutes

18. Cauliflower Rice Burrito Bowl

Health Benefits

- Cauliflower rice is a low-carbohydrate and low-phosphorus alternative.

- Black beans supplies us with plant-based protein and fiber.

- Avocado adds healthy monounsaturated fats.

Ingredients

- 1 head cauliflower, riced

- Black beans of 1 can (15 oz) , drained and rinsed

- Corn kernels (fresh or frozen) of 1 cup

- 1 cup cherry tomatoes, halved

- 1/2 red onion, finely chopped

- 1 avocado, sliced

- Fresh cilantro (for garnish)

- Lime wedges (for serving)

- 1 teaspoon cumin

- 1 teaspoon chili powder

- Salt and pepper to taste

Mode of Preparation

1. In a skillet, sauté riced cauliflower until tender.

2. Add black beans, corn, cherry tomatoes, red onion, cumin, chili powder, salt, and pepper.

3. Cook until heated through, stirring occasionally.

4. Divide the cauliflower mixture into bowls and top with avocado slices, fresh cilantro, and a squeeze of lime.

Nutritional Information

- Calories: 220

- Protein: 10g

- Fiber: 9g

- Potassium: 350mg

- Phosphorus: 160mg

Serving Size: 4

Cooking Time: 20 minutes

Preparation Time: 15 minutes

19. Lemon-Dill Tofu Skewers

Health Benefits

- Tofu provides a versatile, plant-based protein source.

- Lemon and dill add fresh flavors without excess sodium.

- Bell peppers contribute vitamins and antioxidants.

Ingredients

- Firm tofu of 1 block (14 oz), cubed

- 1 lemon, juiced

- 2 tablespoons olive oil

- 2 cloves garlic, minced

- 1 tablespoon fresh dill, chopped

- 1 bell pepper, cut into chunks

- Cherry tomatoes (for skewering)

- Salt and pepper to taste

Mode of Preparation

1. In a bowl, whisk together lemon juice, olive oil, minced garlic, chopped dill, salt, and pepper.

2. Marinate tofu cubes in the mixture for at least 30 minutes.

3. Preheat the grill or grill pan.

4. Thread marinated tofu, bell pepper chunks, and cherry tomatoes onto skewers.

5. Grill skewers until tofu is golden and vegetables are tender, turning occasionally.

6. Serve immediately, optionally with a side of quinoa or a green salad.

Nutritional Information

- Serving Size: 2 skewers

- Calories: 280

- Protein: 14g

- Fiber: 6g

- Potassium: 300mg

- Phosphorus: 150mg

Serving Size: 4

Cooking Time: 15 minutes (plus marination time)

Preparation Time: 45 minutes

CHAPTER 3

Dinner recipes

1.Quinoa and Vegetable Stir-Fry

Health Benefits

- Low in phosphorus and potassium.

- Quinoa provides a complete protein source.

- Abundant in fiber, supporting digestive health.

- Colorful vegetables offer essential vitamins and antioxidants.

Ingredients

- 1 cup quinoa

- 2 cups water

- 1 tablespoon olive oil

- 1 cup broccoli florets

- 1 cup bell peppers, sliced

- 1 cup zucchini, sliced

- 2 cloves garlic, minced

- 2 tablespoons low-sodium soy sauce

- 1 tablespoon fresh ginger, grated

- Salt and pepper to taste

Mode of Preparation

1. Rinse quinoa under cold water.

2. In a saucepan, combine quinoa and water. Bring to a boil, then simmer for 15-20 minutes until water is absorbed.

3. Olive oil should be heated in a large skillet

4. Garlic and ginger should be added, sauté until fragrant.

5. Add broccoli, bell peppers, and zucchini. Stir-fry until vegetables are tender-crisp.

6. Stir in cooked quinoa and soy sauce. Season with salt and pepper.

7. Cook for an additional 5 minutes, ensuring flavors meld.

Nutritional Information

- Calories: 250

- Protein: 9g

- Fiber: 6g

- Potassium: 180mg

- Phosphorus: 150mg

Serving Size: 4

Cooking Time: 25 minutes

Preparation Time: 15 minutes

2: Chickpea and Spinach Curry

Health Benefits

- High in plant-based protein from chickpeas.

- Spinach is a good source of iron and other essential nutrients.

- Low in phosphorus and potassium.

Ingredients

- 2 cans chickpeas, drained and rinsed

- 1 onion, finely chopped

- 2 cloves garlic, minced

- 1 tablespoon olive oil

- 1 can diced tomatoes

- 2 cups fresh spinach

- 1 tablespoon curry powder

- 1 teaspoon turmeric

- 1 teaspoon cumin

- Salt and pepper to taste

- 1 cup water

Mode of Preparation

1. In a large pot, heat olive oil and sauté onion and garlic until translucent.

2. Add curry powder, turmeric, and cumin. Stir until fragrant.

3. Pour in diced tomatoes, chickpeas, and water. Simmer for 15 minutes.

4. Add fresh spinach and cook until wilted.

5. It should be seasoned with salt and pepper to taste.

Nutritional Information

- Calories: 220

- Protein: 10g

- Fiber: 8g

- Potassium: 200mg

- Phosphorus: 160mg

Serving Size: 4

Cooking Time: 25 minutes

Preparation Time: 15 minutes

3: Mushroom and Lentil Stuffed Bell Peppers

Health Benefits

- Lentils provide protein without excess phosphorus.

- Mushrooms offer a savory, meaty texture.

- Low in potassium and sodium.

Ingredients

- 4 large bell peppers, halved

- 1 cup green lentils, cooked

- 1 cup mushrooms, finely chopped

- 1 onion, diced

- 2 cloves garlic, minced

- 1 can crushed tomatoes

- 1 teaspoon oregano

- 1 teaspoon thyme

- Salt and pepper to taste

- 1 tablespoon olive oil

Mode of Preparation

1. Preheat the oven to 375°F (190°C).

2. In a pan, heat olive oil and sauté onions and garlic until softened.

3. Add mushrooms and cook until moisture evaporates.

4. Stir in cooked lentils, crushed tomatoes, oregano, thyme, salt, and pepper.

5. Fill halved bell peppers with the lentil-mushroom mixture.

6. Bake for 25-30 minutes until peppers are tender.

Nutritional Information

- Calories: 180

- Protein: 9g

- Fiber: 7g

- Potassium: 210mg

- Phosphorus: 120mg

Serving Size: 4

Cooking Time: 30 minutes

Preparation Time: 20 minutes

4: Cauliflower and Chickpea Curry Soup

Health Benefits

- Cauliflower is low in phosphorus and potassium

- Chickpeas add plant-based protein.

- Curry spices offer anti-inflammatory properties.

Ingredients

- 1 head cauliflower, chopped

- 1 can chickpeas, drained and rinsed

- 1 onion, diced

- 2 cloves garlic, minced

- 1 can coconut milk

- 1 tablespoon curry powder

- 1 teaspoon cumin

- 1 teaspoon turmeric

- Salt and pepper to taste

- 4 cups vegetable broth

- 1 tablespoon olive oil

Mode of Preparation

1. In a pot, heat olive oil and sauté onions and garlic until translucent.

2. Add cauliflower, chickpeas, curry powder, cumin, and turmeric. Stir to coat.

3. Pour in coconut milk and vegetable broth. Bring to a simmer.

4. Cook until cauliflower is tender, approximately 20 minutes.

5. Season with salt and pepper.

Nutritional Information

- Calories: 220

- Protein: 8g

- Fiber: 6g

- Potassium: 180mg

- Phosphorus: 150mg

Serving Size: 4

Cooking Time: 25 minutes

Preparation Time: 15 minutes

5: Sweet Potato and Black Bean Chili

Health Benefits

- Sweet potatoes provides us with fiber and vitamins.

- Black beans provide plant-based protein.

- Low in sodium and phosphorus.

Ingredients

- 2 sweet potatoes, diced

- 2 cans black beans, drained and rinsed

- 1 onion, diced

- 2 cloves garlic, minced

- 1 can diced tomatoes

- 1 tablespoon chili powder

- 1 teaspoon cumin

- 1 teaspoon paprika

- Salt and pepper to taste

- 4 cups vegetable broth

- 1 tablespoon olive oil

Mode of Preparation

1. In a large pot, heat olive oil and sauté onions and garlic until softened.

2. Add sweet potatoes, black beans, diced tomatoes, chili powder, cumin, and paprika.

3. Pour in vegetable broth and bring to a boil, then simmer for 20-25 minutes.

4. It should be seasoned with salt and pepper to taste.

Nutritional Information

- Calories: 200

- Protein: 7g

- Fiber: 8g

- Potassium: 220mg

- Phosphorus: 130mg

Serving Size: 4

Cooking Time: 30 minutes

Preparation Time: 20 minutes

6: Zucchini Noodles with Tomato and Basil Sauce

Health Benefits

- Zucchini noodles provide a low-carb alternative.

- Tomatoes offer antioxidants and are low in phosphorus.

- Basil adds flavor without sodium.

Ingredients

- 4 medium zucchinis, spiralized

- 1 can diced tomatoes (low-sodium)

- 2 cloves garlic, minced

- 1 tablespoon olive oil

- 1 teaspoon dried basil

- Salt and pepper to taste

- 1/4 cup nutritional yeast (optional)

Mode of Preparation

1. In a pan, heat olive oil and sauté minced garlic until fragrant.

2. Add spiralized zucchini and cook for 3-4 minutes until tender.

3. Pour in diced tomatoes and dried basil. Simmer for an additional 5 minutes.

4. It should be seasoned with salt and pepper to taste.

5. Optionally, sprinkle nutritional yeast for added flavor.

Nutritional Information

- Calories: 80

- Protein: 5g

- Fiber: 4g

- Potassium: 250mg

- Phosphorus: 70mg

Serving Size: 4

Cooking Time: 15 minutes

Preparation Time: 10 minutes

7: Roasted Eggplant and Red Pepper Dip

Health Benefits

- Eggplant is low in potassium and provides fiber.

- Red peppers are rich in vitamins and antioxidants.

- A flavorful dip without excessive sodium.

Ingredients

- 1 large eggplant, diced

- 2 red bell peppers, roasted and chopped

- 2 cloves garlic, minced

- 2 tablespoons tahini

- 2 tablespoons lemon juice

- 1 tablespoon olive oil

- 1 teaspoon cumin

- Salt and pepper to taste

Mode of Preparation

1. Roast red peppers until skin blackens. Peel and chop.

2. In a pan, sauté diced eggplant until tender.

3. In a food processor, combine eggplant, roasted red peppers, minced garlic, tahini, lemon juice, and cumin. Blend until smooth.

4. Drizzle olive oil and season with salt and pepper.

Nutritional Information

- Calories: 40

- Protein: 1g

- Fiber: 2g

- Potassium: 90mg

- Phosphorus: 30mg

Serving Size: 8

Cooking Time: 25 minutes

Preparation Time: 15 minutes

8: Spinach and Artichoke Stuffed Portobello Mushrooms

Health Benefits

- Portobello mushrooms offer a meaty texture and are low in potassium.

- Spinach is rich in iron and low in phosphorus.

- Artichokes add flavor without sodium.

Ingredients

- 4 large portobello mushrooms, stems removed

- 2 cups fresh spinach, chopped

- Artichoke hearts of 1 can, drained and chopped

- 2 cloves garlic, minced

- 1/4 cup nutritional yeast

- 1 tablespoon olive oil

- Salt and pepper to taste

Mode of Preparation

1. Preheat the oven to 375°F (190°C).

2. In a pan, sauté minced garlic in olive oil until fragrant.

3. Add chopped spinach and cook until wilted.

4. Stir in chopped artichoke hearts and nutritional yeast.

5. Fill each portobello mushroom cap with the spinach-artichoke mixture.

6. It should be baked for 20-25 minutes until mushrooms are tender.

Nutritional Information

- Calories: 70

- Protein: 4g

- Fiber: 3g

- Potassium: 150mg

- Phosphorus: 80mg

Serving Size: 4

Cooking Time: 25 minutes

Preparation Time: 15 minutes

9: Lemon Herb Tofu Skewers

Health Benefits

- Tofu provides plant-based protein.

- Lemon and herbs add flavor without sodium.

- Low in potassium and phosphorus.

Ingredients

- 1 block firm tofu, cubed

- Zest and juice of 1 lemon

- 2 tablespoons olive oil

- 2 teaspoons dried thyme

- 1 teaspoon dried rosemary

- 2 cloves garlic, minced

- Salt and pepper to taste

- Wooden skewers, soaked in water

Mode of Preparation

1. In a bowl, mix lemon zest, lemon juice, olive oil, thyme, rosemary, minced garlic, salt, and pepper.

2. Marinate tofu cubes in the mixture for at least 30 minutes.

3. Thread marinated tofu onto soaked wooden skewers.

4. Grill or bake until tofu is golden brown.

Nutritional Information

- Serving Size: 2 skewers

- Calories: 180

- Protein: 12g

- Fiber: 3g

- Potassium: 200mg

- Phosphorus: 100mg

Serving Size: 4

Cooking Time: 15 minutes (plus marination time)
Preparation Time: 10 minutes

10: Cucumber and Avocado Gazpacho

Health Benefits

- Cucumbers provide hydration and are low in potassium.

- Avocado adds healthy fats.

- A refreshing, cold soup perfect for hot days.

Ingredients

- 2 large cucumbers, peeled and diced

- 1 ripe avocado, peeled and pitted

- 1/2 red onion, diced

- 2 cloves garlic, minced

- 2 tablespoons fresh cilantro, chopped

- 3 cups vegetable broth (low-sodium)

- Juice of 2 limes

- Salt and pepper to taste

Mode of Preparation

1. In a blender, combine diced cucumbers, avocado, red onion, minced garlic, cilantro, lime juice, and vegetable broth.

2. Blend until smooth.

3. It should be seasoned with salt and pepper to taste.

4. Leave in the refrigerator for at least 2 hours before serving.

Nutritional Information

- Calories: 90

- Protein: 2g

- Fiber: 4g

- Potassium: 250mg

- Phosphorus: 80mg

Serving Size: 4

Cooking Time: 10 minutes (plus chilling time)

Preparation Time: 15 minutes

11: Mango and Black Bean Salad

Health Benefits

- Black beans offer plant-based protein.

- Mango provides natural sweetness and is low in potassium.

- High fiber content supports digestive health.

Ingredients

- 2 cups black beans, cooked and drained

- 2 ripe mangoes, diced

- 1 red bell pepper, diced

- 1/2 red onion, finely chopped

- 1/4 cup fresh cilantro, chopped

- Juice of 2 limes

- 2 tablespoons olive oil

- Salt and pepper to taste

- Optional: Jalapeño for a spicy kick

Mode of Preparation

1. In a large bowl, combine black beans, diced mangoes, red bell pepper, red onion, and cilantro.

2. In a small bowl, whisk together lime juice, olive oil, salt, and pepper.

3. Dressing should be poured over the salad and toss gently.

4. Add jalapeño if desired for a spicy variation.

Nutritional Information

- Calories: 180

- Protein: 7g

- Fiber: 8g

- Potassium: 250mg

- Phosphorus: 120mg

Serving Size: 4

Preparation Time: 15 minutes

12: Broccoli and Walnut Pesto Pasta

Health Benefits

- Broccoli is low in potassium and phosphorus.

- Walnuts provide heart-healthy fats and protein.

- A flavorful alternative to traditional pesto.

Ingredients

- 2 cups whole wheat pasta, cooked

- 2 cups broccoli florets, steamed

- 1 cup fresh basil leaves

- 1/2 cup walnuts

- 2 cloves garlic, minced

- 1/4 cup nutritional yeast

- Juice of 1 lemon

- 1/4 cup olive oil

- Salt and pepper to taste

Mode of Preparation

1. In a food processor, combine broccoli, basil, walnuts, minced garlic, nutritional yeast, and lemon juice.

2. Pulse until ingredients are finely chopped.

3. With the processor running, slowly add olive oil until a smooth pesto consistency is reached.

4. It should be seasoned with salt and pepper to taste.

5. Toss the pesto with cooked pasta and serve.

Nutritional Information

- Calories: 320

- Protein: 12g

- Fiber: 8g

- Potassium: 200mg

- Phosphorus: 150mg

Serving Size: 4

Cooking Time: 20 minutes

Preparation Time: 15 minutes

13: Crispy Tofu and Asparagus Stir-Fry

Health Benefits

- Tofu offers a plant-based protein source.

- Asparagus is low in potassium and high in fiber.

- Stir-frying retains nutrients without excessive fats.

Ingredients

- Extra-firm tofu of 1 block, pressed and cubed

- 1 bunch asparagus, trimmed and cut into bite-sized pieces

- 1 red bell pepper, sliced

- 2 tablespoons soy sauce (low-sodium)

- 1 tablespoon hoisin sauce

- 1 tablespoon sesame oil

- 2 tablespoons cornstarch

- 2 tablespoons vegetable oil

- 2 cloves garlic, minced

- 1 tablespoon ginger, grated

- Sesame seeds for garnish

Mode of Preparation

1. Toss cubed tofu in cornstarch until coated.

2. Heat vegetable oil in a pan and fry tofu until golden brown. Set aside.

3. In the same pan, sauté garlic and ginger until fragrant.

4. Add asparagus and red bell pepper. Stir-fry until vegetables are tender-crisp.

5. Return the crispy tofu to the pan.

6. Mix in soy sauce, hoisin sauce, and sesame oil.

7. Garnish with sesame seeds before serving.

Nutritional Information

- Calories: 250

- Protein: 12g

- Fiber: 5g

- Potassium: 280mg

- Phosphorus: 160mg

Serving Size: 4

Cooking Time: 25 minutes

Preparation Time: 20 minutes

14: Cauliflower Rice and Black-Eyed Pea Pilaf

Health Benefits

- Cauliflower rice is a low-carb, low-phosphorus alternative.

- Black-eyed peas provide plant-based protein.

- Rich in fiber and essential nutrients.

Ingredients

- 1 head cauliflower, riced

- 1 can black-eyed peas, drained and rinsed

- 1 onion, finely chopped

- 2 cloves garlic, minced

- 1/2 cup cherry tomatoes, halved

- 1/4 cup fresh parsley, chopped

- 1 tablespoon olive oil

- 1 teaspoon cumin

- Salt and pepper to taste

Mode of Preparation

1. In a pan, sauté chopped onion and minced garlic in olive oil until softened.

2. Cauliflower rice should be added and cook until tender.

3. Stir in black-eyed peas, cherry tomatoes, cumin, salt, and pepper.

4. Cook for an additional 5 minutes until ingredients are well combined.

5. Garnish with fresh parsley before serving.

Nutritional Information

- Calories: 180

- Protein: 8g

- Fiber: 6g

- Potassium: 220mg

- Phosphorus: 130mg

Serving Size: 4

Cooking Time: 20 minutes

Preparation Time: 15 minutes

15: Cabbage and Lentil Stew

Health Benefits

- Lentils offer plant-based protein.

- Cabbage is excellently low in potassium and phosphorus.

- A hearty and satisfying stew rich in fiber.

Ingredients

- Green or brown lentils of 1 Cup, rinsed

- 1 small cabbage, shredded

- 2 carrots, diced

- 1 onion, finely chopped

- 2 cloves garlic, minced

- 1 can diced tomatoes (low-sodium)

- 4 cups vegetable broth

- 1 teaspoon smoked paprika

- 1 teaspoon dried thyme

- Salt and pepper to taste

- 1 tablespoon olive oil

Mode of Preparation

1. In a large pot, heat olive oil and sauté onion and garlic until softened.

2. Add carrots, cabbage, lentils, diced tomatoes, vegetable broth, smoked paprika, and dried thyme.

3. Bring to a boil, then simmer for 30-40 minutes until lentils are tender.

4. It should be seasoned with salt and pepper to taste.

Nutritional Information

- Calories: 220

- Protein: 12g

- Fiber: 10g

- Potassium: 280mg

- Phosphorus: 150mg

Serving Size: 4

Cooking Time: 45 minutes

Preparation Time: 15 minutes

16: Brussels Sprouts and Pomegranate Salad

Health Benefits

- Brussels sprouts are low in potassium and phosphorus.

- Pomegranate seeds offer antioxidants and a burst of sweetness.

- A crunchy and flavorful salad.

Ingredients

- 2 cups Brussels sprouts, shaved

- 1/2 cup pomegranate seeds

- 1/4 cup walnuts, chopped

- 1/4 cup vegan feta cheese, crumbled

- 2 tablespoons balsamic vinegar

- 1 tablespoon olive oil

- Salt and pepper to taste

Mode of Preparation

1. Shave Brussels sprouts using a knife or mandoline.

2. In a bowl, combine shaved Brussels sprouts, pomegranate seeds, chopped walnuts, and crumbled vegan feta.

3. Whisk together balsamic vinegar, olive oil, salt, and pepper in a small bowl,

4. The dressing should be drizzle over the salad and toss gently.

Nutritional Information

- Calories: 180

- Protein: 6g

- Fiber: 7g

- Potassium: 220mg

- Phosphorus: 120mg

Serving Size: 4

Preparation Time: 15 minutes

17: Stuffed Acorn Squash with Quinoa and Cranberries

Health Benefits

- Acorn squash is rich in vitamins and low in potassium.

- Quinoa provides a complete protein source.

- Cranberries serves as a sweetness and antioxidants.

Ingredients

- Halved 2 acorn squash with the seeds removed

- 1 cup quinoa, cooked

- 1/2 cup dried cranberries

- 1/4 cup pecans, chopped

- 2 tablespoons maple syrup

- 1 teaspoon cinnamon

- Salt and pepper to taste

- 1 tablespoon olive oil

Mode of Preparation

1. Preheat the oven to 400°F (200°C).

2. Brush the cut sides of acorn squash with olive oil and sprinkle with salt and pepper.

3. Roast squash in the oven for 30-40 minutes until tender.

4. In a bowl, mix cooked quinoa, dried cranberries, chopped pecans, maple syrup, and cinnamon.

5. Spoon the quinoa mixture into the roasted acorn squash halves.

Nutritional Information

- Calories: 250

- Protein: 6g

- Fiber: 7g

- Potassium: 320mg

- Phosphorus: 140mg

Serving Size: 4

Cooking Time: 45 minutes

Preparation Time: 20 minutes

18: Lemon Herb Roasted Chickpeas

Health Benefits

- Chickpeas offer plant-based protein.

- Lemon and herbs add flavor without sodium.

- A crunchy and satisfying snack or salad topper.

Ingredients

- 2 cans chickpeas, drained and rinsed

- Zest and juice of 2 lemons

- 2 tablespoons olive oil

- 1 teaspoon dried thyme

- 1 teaspoon dried rosemary

- 1 teaspoon garlic powder

- Salt and pepper to taste

Mode of Preparation

1. Preheat the oven to 400°F (200°C).

2. Pat chickpeas dry with a paper towel.

3. In a bowl, toss chickpeas with lemon zest, lemon juice, olive oil, thyme, rosemary, garlic powder, salt, and pepper.

4. Chickpeas should be spread on a baking sheet in a single layer.

5. Roast for 25-30 minutes until golden and crispy.

Nutritional Information

- Calories: 180

- Protein: 8g

- Fiber: 6g

- Potassium: 220mg

- Phosphorus: 150mg

Serving Size: 4

Cooking Time: 30 minutes

Preparation Time: 10 minutes

CHAPTER 4

Snacks and Appetizer

1: Avocado and Tomato Bruschetta

Health Benefits

- Rich in heart-healthy fats from avocados.

- Tomatoes provide antioxidants and are low in potassium.

- Whole-grain bread provides fiber for digestive health.

Ingredients

- 1 ripe avocado, diced

- 2 tomatoes, diced

- 1 clove garlic, minced

- 2 tablespoons red onion, finely chopped

- 1 tablespoon fresh basil, chopped

- 1 tablespoon balsamic vinegar

- Salt and pepper to taste

- 4 slices whole-grain baguette

Mode of Preparation

1. In a bowl, combine diced avocado, tomatoes, garlic, red onion, and basil.

2. Add balsamic vinegar, salt, and pepper. Mix gently.

3. Toast whole-grain baguette slices until golden brown.

4. Spoon avocado-tomato mixture onto the toasted baguette.

Nutritional Information

- Calories: 120

- Protein: 3g

- Fiber: 5g

- Potassium: 200mg

- Phosphorus: 80mg

Serving Size: 2 slices

Cooking Time: 10 minutes

Preparation Time: 15 minutes

2: Sweet Potato and Kale Bites
Health Benefits

- Sweet potatoes offer fiber and are low in potassium.

- Kale is rich in vitamins and minerals, including iron and calcium.

- Plant-based protein from chickpea flour.

Ingredients

- 2 medium sweet potatoes, grated

- 2 cups kale, finely chopped

- 1 cup chickpea flour

- 1/2 cup nutritional yeast

- 1 teaspoon garlic powder

- 1 teaspoon onion powder

- Salt and pepper to taste

- 2 tablespoons olive oil

Mode of Preparation

1. Preheat oven to 375°F (190°C).

2. In a bowl, combine grated sweet potatoes, chopped kale, chickpea flour, nutritional yeast, garlic powder, onion powder, salt, and pepper.

3. Form mixture into bite-sized balls and place on a baking sheet.

4. Drizzle olive oil over the bites and bake for 20-25 minutes until golden brown.

Nutritional Information

- Calories: 150

- Protein: 6g

- Fiber: 4g

- Potassium: 180mg

- Phosphorus: 90mg

Serving Size: 4 bites

Cooking Time: 25 minutes

Preparation Time: 15 minutes

3: Cucumber and Chickpea Salad Cups

Health Benefits

- Cucumbers are low in potassium.

- Chickpeas provide plant-based protein and fiber.

- Fresh herbs add antioxidants and flavor.

Ingredients

- 2 cucumbers, sliced into rounds

- 1 can (15 oz) chickpeas, drained and rinsed

- 1/2 cup cherry tomatoes, halved

- 1/4 cup red onion, finely chopped

- 2 tablespoons fresh parsley, chopped

- 1 tablespoon olive oil

- 1 tablespoon lemon juice

- Salt and pepper to taste

Mode of Preparation

1. In a bowl, mix chickpeas, cherry tomatoes, red onion, parsley, olive oil, lemon juice, salt, and pepper.

2. Scoop out the center of cucumber rounds to create cups.

3. Fill cucumber cups with the chickpea salad.

Nutritional Information

- Calories: 160

- Protein: 7g

- Fiber: 5g

- Potassium: 220mg

- Phosphorus: 100mg

Serving Size: 6 cups

Cooking Time: 10 minutes

Preparation Time: 15 minutes

4: Quinoa and Black Bean Stuffed Peppers

Health Benefits

- Quinoa provides complete protein and is low in potassium.

- Black beans provides with plant-based protein and fiber

- Bell peppers gives us vitamins A and C.

Ingredients

- Halved 4 bell pepper after the seed has been removed

- 1 cup cooked quinoa

- Black beans of 1 can (15 oz) , drained and rinsed

- 1 cup corn kernels

- 1 cup diced tomatoes

- 1/2 cup red onion, finely chopped

- 1 teaspoon cumin

- 1 teaspoon chili powder

- Salt and pepper to taste

Mode of Preparation

1. Preheat oven to 375°F (190°C).

2. In a bowl, mix cooked quinoa, black beans, corn, tomatoes, red onion, cumin, chili powder, salt, and pepper.

3. Stuff bell pepper halves with the quinoa and black bean mixture.

4. Bake for 25-30 minutes until peppers are tender.

Nutritional Information

- Calories: 220

- Protein: 9g

- Fiber: 8g

- Potassium: 250mg

- Phosphorus: 120mg

Serving Size: 2 halves

Cooking Time: 30 minutes

Preparation Time: 20 minutes

5: Zucchini and Hummus Roll-Ups

Health Benefits

- Zucchini is low in potassium and adds a crisp texture.

- Hummus is rich in plant-based protein and healthy fats.

- Fresh herbs contribute antioxidants and flavor.

Ingredients

- 2 large zucchinis, thinly sliced lengthwise

- 1 cup hummus (store-bought or homemade)

- 1/4 cup sun-dried tomatoes, chopped

- 2 tablespoons fresh basil, chopped

- 1 tablespoon pine nuts

- Salt and pepper to taste

Mode of Preparation

1. Lay out zucchini slices and spread hummus evenly on each slice.

2. Sprinkle sun-dried tomatoes, fresh basil, and pine nuts on top.

3. Roll up the zucchini slices and secure with toothpicks.

4. Chill in the refrigerator for 15-20 minutes before serving.

Nutritional Information

- Calories: 180

- Protein: 6g

- Fiber: 5g

- Potassium: 180mg

- Phosphorus: 100mg

Serving Size: 4 roll-ups

Preparation Time: 15 minutes

6: Mango Salsa with Baked Plantain Chips

Health Benefits

- Mangoes provide vitamins A and C.

- Plantains provides us with complex carbohydrates.

- Fresh cilantro adds antioxidants and flavor.

Ingredients

- 2 ripe mangoes, diced

- 1 cup red bell pepper, finely chopped

- 1/2 cup red onion, finely chopped

- 1/4 cup fresh cilantro, chopped

- 1 tablespoon lime juice

- Salt and pepper to taste

- 2 large green plantains

Mode of Preparation

1. Preheat oven to 375°F (190°C).

2. In a bowl, combine diced mangoes, red bell pepper, red onion, cilantro, lime juice, salt, and pepper.

3. Peel plantains and slice thinly.

4. Arrange plantain slices on a baking sheet and bake for 15-20 minutes until golden brown.

5. Serve plantain chips with mango salsa.

Nutritional Information

- Calories: 160

- Protein: 2g

- Fiber: 4g

- Potassium: 220mg

- Phosphorus: 80mg

Serving Size: 1 cup salsa with 1 cup plantain chips

Cooking Time: 20 minutes

Preparation Time: 15 minutes

7: Cauliflower Buffalo Bites

Health Benefits

- Cauliflower is low in potassium and provides vitamins C and K.

- Almond flour adds a gluten-free alternative to traditional breading.

- Buffalo sauce offers a spicy kick without excessive sodium.

Ingredients

- 1 medium cauliflower head, cut into florets

- 1 cup almond flour

- 1 teaspoon garlic powder

- 1 teaspoon smoked paprika

- 1/2 cup unsweetened almond milk

- 1/2 cup buffalo sauce

- 1 tablespoon olive oil

- Green onions for garnish (optional)

Mode of Preparation

1. Preheat oven to 450°F (230°C).

2. In a bowl, combine almond flour, garlic powder, and smoked paprika.

3. Dip cauliflower florets in almond milk, then coat in the almond flour mixture.

4. Arrange on a baking sheet, drizzle with olive oil, and bake for 20-25 minutes.

5. Toss baked cauliflower in buffalo sauce and garnish with green onions if desired.

Nutritional Information

- Calories: 180

- Protein: 6g

- Fiber: 4g

- Potassium: 250mg

- Phosphorus: 100mg

Serving Size: 1 cup

Cooking Time: 25 minutes

Preparation Time: 15 minutes

8: Spinach and Artichoke Dip with Veggie Sticks

Health Benefits

- Spinach supplies of iron and vitamins.

- Artichokes provide dietary fiber and are low in potassium.

- Veggie sticks add crunch and essential nutrients.

Ingredients

- 2 cups fresh spinach, chopped

- Artichoke hearts of 1 can (14 oz), drained and chopped

- 1 cup vegan cream cheese

- 1/2 cup nutritional yeast

- 1/4 cup almond milk

- 2 cloves garlic, minced

- Salt and pepper to taste

- Carrot and cucumber sticks for dipping

Mode of Preparation

1. In a saucepan, sauté chopped spinach until wilted.

2. Add artichoke hearts, vegan cream cheese, nutritional yeast, almond milk, garlic, salt, and pepper.

3. Mix thoroughly until well combined and heated through.

4. Serve with carrot and cucumber sticks.

Nutritional Information

- Calories: 120

- Protein: 4g

- Fiber: 3g

- Potassium: 180mg

- Phosphorus: 80mg

Serving Size: 1/4 cup dip with 1 cup veggie sticks

Cooking Time: 15 minutes

Preparation Time: 10 minutes

9: Chia Pudding Parfait with Mixed Berries

Health Benefits

- Chia seeds is an excellent source of omega-3 fatty acids and fiber.

- Mixed berries offer antioxidants and vitamins.

- Coconut yogurt adds a dairy-free alternative with a creamy texture.

Ingredients

- 1/4 cup chia seeds

- 1 cup unsweetened almond milk

- 1 teaspoon vanilla extract

- 2 tablespoons maple syrup

- Mixed berries of 1 Cup (strawberries, blueberries, raspberries)

- 1 cup coconut yogurt

Mode of Preparation

1. Mix chia seeds, almond milk, vanilla extract, and maple syrup in a bowl

2. Refrigerate for at least 2 hours or overnight until a pudding-like consistency is achieved.

3. In a glass or jar, layer chia pudding with mixed berries and coconut yogurt.

4. Repeat layers and top with additional berries.

Nutritional Information

- Calories: 220

- Protein: 6g

- Fiber: 12g

- Potassium: 200mg

- Phosphorus: 120mg

Serving Size: 1 parfait

Cooking Time: 2 hours (for chia pudding setting)

Preparation Time: 15 minutes

10: Lemon-Herb Marinated Grilled Tofu Skewers

Health Benefits

- Tofu provides plant-based protein and is low in potassium.

- Lemon and herbs add flavor without excess sodium.

- Grilling enhances the smoky taste with minimal added fats.

Ingredients

- Extra-firm tofu of 1 block, pressed and cut into cubes

- 2 tablespoons olive oil

- Zest and juice of 1 lemon

- 2 cloves garlic, minced

- 1 tablespoon fresh rosemary, chopped

- 1 tablespoon fresh thyme, chopped

- Salt and pepper to taste

- Cherry tomatoes and bell pepper chunks for skewering

Mode of Preparation

1. In a bowl, whisk together olive oil, lemon zest, lemon juice, garlic, rosemary, thyme, salt, and pepper.

2. Marinate tofu cubes in the mixture for at least 30 minutes.

3. Skewer marinated tofu, cherry tomatoes, and bell pepper chunks.

4. Grill skewers until tofu is golden and vegetables are tender.

Nutritional Information

- Calories: 180

- Protein: 12g

- Fiber: 3g

- Potassium: 220mg

- Phosphorus: 160mg

Serving Size: 2 skewers

Cooking Time: 15 minutes

Preparation Time: 45 minutes (including marination

CHAPTER 5

Desserts

1: Chia Seed Pudding with Mixed Berries

Health Benefits

- Rich in fiber for digestive health.

- Low in potassium, suitable for CKD Stage 5 patients.

- Packed with antioxidants from mixed berries.

Ingredients

- 1/4 cup chia seeds

- 1 cup unsweetened almond milk

- 1 tablespoon maple syrup

- 1/2 teaspoon vanilla extract

- Mixed berries (strawberries, blueberries, raspberries) of 1/2 cup

Mode of Preparation

1. In a bowl, mix chia seeds, almond milk, maple syrup, and vanilla extract.

2. Mix well and refrigerate for at least 4 hours or overnight.

3. Before serving, top with mixed berries.

Nutritional Information (per serving)

- Calories: 180

- Protein: 4g

- Fiber: 10g

- Potassium: 120mg

Serving Size: 1 cup

Cooking Time: 4 hours (chilling time)

Preparation Time: 5 minutes

2: Avocado Chocolate Mousse

Health Benefits

- Heart-healthy monounsaturated fats from avocados.

- Low in potassium and phosphorus, suitable for CKD Stage 5 patients.

- Rich in antioxidants from cocoa.

Ingredients

- 2 ripe avocados

- 1/4 cup unsweetened cocoa powder

- 1/4 cup maple syrup

- 1 teaspoon vanilla extract

- Pinch of salt

Mode of Preparation

1. Blend avocados, cocoa powder, maple syrup, vanilla extract, and salt until smooth.

2. Refrigerate for at least 2 hours before serving.

Nutritional Information (per serving):

- Calories: 200

- Protein: 3g

- Fiber: 8g

- Potassium: 250mg

Serving Size: 1/2 cup

Cooking Time: 2 hours (chilling time)

Preparation Time: 10 minutes

3: Baked Apple Cinnamon Oatmeal Cups

Health Benefits

- Oats provide soluble fiber for heart health.

- Low in potassium and phosphorus, suitable for CKD Stage 5 patients.

- Apples offer antioxidants and natural sweetness.

Ingredients

- 2 cups rolled oats

- 1 teaspoon cinnamon

- 1/2 teaspoon baking powder

- 1/4 cup maple syrup

- 1 1/2 cups unsweetened almond milk

- 1 medium apple, diced

Mode of Preparation

1. Preheat oven to 350°F (175°C).

2. In a bowl, mix oats, cinnamon, baking powder, maple syrup, and almond milk.

3. Fold in diced apples.

4. Mixture should be spooned into a greased muffin tin.

5. It should be baked for 25-30 minutes or until golden brown.

Nutritional Information (per serving)

- Calories: 180
- Protein: 5g
- Fiber: 4g
- Potassium: 150mg

Serving Size: 2 oatmeal cups

Cooking Time: 30 minutes

Preparation Time: 10 minutes

4: Coconut Rice Pudding with Mango

Health Benefits

- Coconut milk adds richness without dairy.

- Low in potassium, suitable for CKD Stage 5 patients.

- Mango provides vitamins and natural sweetness.

Ingredients

- 1 cup arborio rice

- 2 cups light coconut milk

- 1/4 cup maple syrup

- 1 teaspoon vanilla extract

- 1 ripe mango, diced

Mode of Preparation

1. In a saucepan, combine rice, coconut milk, maple syrup, and vanilla extract.

2. Bring to a simmer and cook until rice is tender.

3. Allow to cool, then refrigerate for at least 2 hours.

4. Top with diced mango before serving.

Nutritional Information (per serving)

- Calories: 220

- Protein: 3g

- Fiber: 2g

- Potassium: 100mg

Serving Size: 1/2 cup

Cooking Time: 30 minutes

Preparation Time: 10 minutes

5: Sweet Potato and Walnut Cookies

Health Benefits

- Sweet potatoes are rich in fiber, vitamins, and antioxidants.

- Walnuts provide omega-3 fatty acids and added texture.

- Low in potassium and phosphorus, suitable for CKD Stage 5 patients.

Ingredients

- 1 cup mashed sweet potatoes

- 1/2 cup almond flour

- 1/4 cup maple syrup

- 1 teaspoon cinnamon

- 1/2 cup chopped walnuts

Mode of Preparation

1. Preheat oven to 350°F (175°C).

2. In a bowl, mix mashed sweet potatoes, almond flour, maple syrup, and cinnamon.

3. Fold in chopped walnuts.

4. Spoon onto a lined baking sheet and flatten with a fork.

5. It should be baked for 20 minutes or until edges are golden.

Nutritional Information (per serving)

- Calories: 160

- Protein: 3g

- Fiber: 2g

- Potassium: 120mg

Serving Size: 2 cookies

Cooking Time: 20 minutes

Preparation Time: 15 minutes

6: Blueberry Almond Oat Bars

Health Benefits

- Oats provide fiber for digestive health.

- Almonds offer healthy fats and added crunch.

- Blueberries are rich in antioxidants and low in potassium.

Ingredients

- 2 cups rolled oats

- 1 cup almond flour

- 1/4 cup maple syrup

- 1/2 cup almond butter

- 1/2 teaspoon almond extract

- 1 cup fresh or frozen blueberries

Mode of Preparation

1. Preheat oven to 350°F (175°C) and line a baking dish with parchment paper.

2. In a bowl, combine oats, almond flour, maple syrup, almond butter, and almond extract.

3. Press half of the mixture into the prepared baking dish.

4. Sprinkle blueberries evenly over the mixture.

5. Crumble the remaining oat mixture over the top.

6. It should be baked for 25-30 minutes or until golden brown.

Nutritional Information (per serving)

- Calories: 210

- Protein: 6g

- Fiber: 4g

- Potassium: 100mg

Serving Size: 1 bar

Cooking Time: 30 minutes

Preparation Time: 15 minutes

7: Cinnamon Walnut Baked Apples

Health Benefits

- Apples provide fiber and natural sweetness.

- Walnuts offer omega-3 fatty acids and added texture.

- Cinnamon adds flavor without sodium.

Ingredients

- 4 large apples, cored

- 1/2 cup chopped walnuts

- 2 tablespoons maple syrup

- 1 teaspoon ground cinnamon

- 1/2 teaspoon vanilla extract

Mode of Preparation

1. Preheat oven to 375°F (190°C).

2. In a bowl, mix chopped walnuts, maple syrup, cinnamon, and vanilla extract.

3. Stuff each cored apple with the walnut mixture.

4. Place apples in a baking dish and bake for 25-30 minutes or until tender.

Nutritional Information (per serving)

- Calories: 180

- Protein: 2g

- Fiber: 6g

- Potassium: 150mg

Serving Size: 1 baked apple

Cooking Time: 30 minutes

Preparation Time: 15 minutes

8: Pumpkin Chia Seed Muffins

Health Benefits

- Pumpkin is a good sources of fiber, vitamins, and antioxidants.

- Chia seeds add omega-3 fatty acids and texture.

- Low in potassium and suitable for CKD Stage 5 patients.

Ingredients

- 1 cup canned pumpkin puree

- 1/4 cup chia seeds

- 1/4 cup maple syrup

- 1 teaspoon pumpkin pie spice

- 1 1/2 cups whole wheat flour

- 1/2 teaspoon baking soda

Mode of Preparation

1. Preheat oven to 375°F (190°C) and line a muffin tin with paper liners.

2. In a bowl, mix pumpkin puree, chia seeds, maple syrup, and pumpkin pie spice.

3. In a separate bowl, combine whole wheat flour and baking soda.

4. Wet ingredients should be added and stir until just combined.

5. Spoon the batter into the muffin tin and bake for 20-25 minutes.

Nutritional Information (per serving)

- Calories: 150

- Protein: 4g

- Fiber: 5g

- Potassium: 100mg

Serving Size: 1 muffin

Cooking Time: 25 minutes

Preparation Time: 10 minutes

9: Mango Sorbet

Health Benefits

- Mangoes offer vitamins, minerals, and antioxidants.

- A refreshing and low-potassium dessert suitable for CKD Stage 5 patients.

Ingredients

- 2 ripe mangoes, peeled and diced

- 2 tablespoons maple syrup

- 1 tablespoon lime juice

- 1/2 cup water

Mode of Preparation

1. Place diced mangoes in a blender or food processor.

2. Add maple syrup, lime juice, and water.

3. Blend until smooth.

4. Pour the mixture into a shallow dish and freeze for at least 4 hours, stirring every hour.

Nutritional Information (per serving)

- Calories: 120

- Protein: 1g

- Fiber: 2g

- Potassium: 150mg

Serving Size: 1/2 cup

Cooking Time: 4 hours (freezing time)

Preparation Time: 10 minutes

10: Raspberry Almond Chia Jam

Health Benefits

- Raspberries are good source of antioxidants and low in potassium.

- Chia seeds add omega-3 fatty acids and help thicken the jam.

- A versatile topping for various desserts.

Ingredients

- 2 cups fresh or frozen raspberries

- 2 tablespoons chia seeds

- 2 tablespoons maple syrup

- 1/2 teaspoon almond extract

Mode of Preparation

1. In a saucepan, combine raspberries and maple syrup.

2. Cook over medium heat until raspberries break down.

3. Remove from heat and stir in chia seeds and almond extract.

4. Serve after refrigerating Let it cool, for at least 2 hours.

Nutritional Information (per serving)

- Calories: 50

- Protein: 1g

- Fiber: 5g

- Potassium: 80mg

Serving Size: 1 tablespoon

Cooking Time: 15 minutes

Preparation Time: 5 minutes

CHAPTER 6

Beverages

1. Berry Citrus Smoothie

Health Benefits

- Rich in antioxidants, supporting kidney health.

- Low in potassium and phosphorus, suitable for CKD Stage 5.

- Provides hydration and essential vitamins.

Ingredients

- Mixed berries of 1 cup (strawberries, blueberries, raspberries)

- 1/2 banana (sliced and frozen)

- 1/2 cup orange juice (unsweetened)

- Water or almond milk of 1/2 cup (unsweetened)

- 1 tablespoon chia seeds (optional)

Mode of Preparation

1. Combine berries, frozen banana, orange juice, and water or almond milk in a blender.

2. Blend until smooth.

3. Stir in chia seeds for added fiber and omega-3s (optional).

4. Pour into a glass and enjoy!

Nutritional Information

- Calories: 150

- Protein: 3g

- Fiber: 7g

- Potassium: 180mg

- Phosphorus: 80mg

Serving Size: 1 glass

Cooking Time: 5 minutes

Preparation Time: 5 minutes

2. Cucumber Mint Cooler

Health Benefits

- Excellent for hydration without excess potassium.

- Contains anti-inflammatory properties from fresh mint.

- Low in phosphorus, suitable for CKD patients.

Ingredients

- 1 cucumber (peeled and sliced)

- 1/4 cup fresh mint leaves

- 1 tablespoon lime juice

- 1 teaspoon agave syrup (optional)

- 2 cups ice cubes

Mode of Preparation

1. Blend cucumber, mint leaves, lime juice, and agave syrup until smooth.

2. Strain the mixture to remove pulp.

3. Pour over ice cubes and garnish with mint leaves.

Nutritional Information

- Calories: 25

- Protein: 1g

- Fiber: 2g

- Potassium: 150mg

- Phosphorus: 40mg

Serving Size: 1 glass

Cooking Time: 10 minutes (including blending)

Preparation Time: 5 minutes

3. Ginger Turmeric Tea

Health Benefits

- Anti-inflammatory properties from ginger and turmeric.

- Low in potassium and phosphorus.

- Aids digestion and supports immune function.

Ingredients

- 1 tablespoon fresh ginger (grated)

- 1/2 teaspoon ground turmeric

- 1 tablespoon lemon juice

- 1 teaspoon agave syrup (optional)

- 2 cups hot water

Mode of Preparation

1. In a teapot, combine grated ginger, ground turmeric, lemon juice, and agave syrup.

2. Pour hot water over the mixture and steep for 5 minutes.

3. Strain into a cup and serve.

Nutritional Information

- Calories: 15

- Protein: 0.5g

- Fiber: 0.5g

- Potassium: 50mg

- Phosphorus: 20mg

Serving Size: 1 cup

Cooking Time: 5 minutes

Preparation Time: 10 minutes (including steeping)

4. Hibiscus Berry Iced Tea

Health Benefits

- Hibiscus helps to lower blood pressure.

- Berries add antioxidants and flavor.

- Low in potassium and phosphorus.

Ingredients

- 2 hibiscus tea bags

- 1 cup mixed berries (fresh or frozen)

- 1 tablespoon agave syrup (optional)

- 2 cups boiling water

- Ice cubes

Mode of Preparation

1. Steep hibiscus tea bags in boiling water for 10 minutes.

2. Tea bags should be removed and let the tea cool.

3. Blend mixed berries and agave syrup until smooth.

4. Mix berry puree with hibiscus tea.

5. Serve over ice cubes.

Nutritional Information

- Calories: 30

- Protein: 0.5g

- Fiber: 3g

- Potassium: 70mg

- Phosphorus: 20mg

Serving Size: 1 glass

Cooking Time: 15 minutes (including steeping and blending)

Preparation Time: 10 minutes

5. Minty Green Tea Lemonade

Health Benefits

- Green tea is rich in antioxidants.

- Mint aids digestion and adds a refreshing flavor.

- Low in potassium and phosphorus.

Ingredients

- 2 green tea bags

- 1 tablespoon fresh mint leaves

- 1 tablespoon lemon juice

- 1 teaspoon agave syrup (optional)

- 2 cups boiling water

- Ice cubes

Mode of Preparation

1. Steep green tea bags and mint leaves in boiling water for 5 minutes.

2. Remove tea bags and mint leaves; let the tea cool.

3. Stir in lemon juice and agave syrup.

4.   Serve over ice cubes.

Nutritional Information

- Calories: 15

- Protein: 0.5g

- Fiber: 0.5g

- Potassium: 30mg

- Phosphorus: 10mg

Serving Size: 1 glass

Cooking Time: 10 minutes (including steeping)

Preparation Time: 5 minutes

6. Golden Milk Latte

Health Benefits

- Turmeric provides anti-inflammatory properties.

- Black pepper enhances curcumin absorption.

- Low in potassium and phosphorus.

Ingredients

- 1 cup unsweetened almond milk

- 1/2 teaspoon ground turmeric

- 1/4 teaspoon ground cinnamon

- Pinch of black pepper

- 1 teaspoon agave syrup (optional)

Mode of Preparation

1. Almond milk should be heated in a small saucepan over medium heat.

2. Add turmeric, cinnamon, black pepper, and agave syrup.

3. Whisk continuously until well combined and heated
    through.

4. Pour into a mug and enjoy the warm, comforting
    drink.

Nutritional Information

- Calories: 30

- Protein: 1g

- Fiber: 1g

- Potassium: 50mg

- Phosphorus: 20mg

Serving Size: 1 cup

Cooking Time: 5 minutes

Preparation Time: 5 minutes

7. Chia Seed Lemonade

Health Benefits

- Chia seeds provides with fiber and omega-3 fatty acids.

- Lemon provides a refreshing, citrusy flavor.

- Low in potassium and phosphorus.

Ingredients

- 2 tablespoons chia seeds

- 1/4 cup fresh lemon juice

- 1 tablespoon agave syrup

- 2 cups cold water

- Ice cubes

Mode of Preparation

1. Mix chia seeds and lemon juice in a glass; let it sit for 10 minutes.

2. Stir in agave syrup.

3. Add cold water and ice cubes; stir well.

4. Allow chia seeds to expand and thicken the lemonade.

5. Serve chilled.

Nutritional Information

- Calories: 50

- Protein: 1g

- Fiber: 6g

- Potassium: 70mg

- Phosphorus: 40mg

Serving Size: 1 glass

Cooking Time: 10 minutes (including soaking time)

Preparation Time: 15 minutes

8. Refreshing Cucumber Basil Cooler

Health Benefits

- Cucumber is hydrating and low in potassium.

- Basil adds a burst of flavor and anti-inflammatory properties.

- Low in potassium and phosphorus.

Ingredients

- 1 cucumber (sliced)

- 1/4 cup fresh basil leaves

- 1 tablespoon lime juice

- 1 teaspoon agave syrup (optional)

- 2 cups cold water

- Ice cubes

Mode of Preparation

1. In a pitcher, combine cucumber slices, basil leaves, lime juice, and agave syrup.

2. Muddle the ingredients to release flavors.

3. Add cold water and stir well.

4. Refrigerate for at least 30 minutes.

5. Serve over ice cubes.

Nutritional Information

- Calories: 20

- Protein: 1g

- Fiber: 1.5g

- Potassium: 60mg

- Phosphorus: 30mg

Serving Size: 1 glass

Cooking Time: 5 minutes

Preparation Time: 35 minutes (including chilling time)

9. Pineapple Mint Smoothie

Health Benefits

- Pineapple is a low-potassium, vitamin C-rich fruit.

- Mint aids digestion and adds a refreshing element.

- Low in potassium and phosphorus.

Ingredients

- 1 cup fresh pineapple chunks

- 1/2 cup fresh mint leaves

- 1/2 banana (sliced and frozen)

- 1/2 cup coconut water (unsweetened)

- 1/2 cup water

- 1 tablespoon flaxseeds (optional)

Mode of Preparation

1. Blend pineapple chunks, mint leaves, frozen banana, coconut water, and water until smooth.

2. Stir in flaxseeds for added fiber and omega-3s (optional).

3. Turn into a glass and enjoy the tropical goodness.

Nutritional Information

- Calories: 120

- Protein: 2g

- Fiber: 4g

- Potassium: 170mg

- Phosphorus: 60mg

Serving Size: 1 glass

Cooking Time: 5 minutes

Preparation Time: 5 minutes

10. Cherry Almond Milkshake

Health Benefits

- Cherries provide antioxidants and are low in potassium.

- Almond milk adds creaminess without excessive phosphorus.

- Low in potassium and phosphorus.

Ingredients

- 1 cup frozen cherries

- 1 cup unsweetened almond milk

- 1/4 teaspoon almond extract

- 1 tablespoon almond butter

- 1 teaspoon agave syrup (optional)

Mode of Preparation

1. Blend frozen cherries, almond milk, almond extract, almond butter, and agave syrup until smooth.

2. Pour into a glass and savor the delightful milkshake.

Nutritional Information

- Calories: 150

- Protein: 3g

- Fiber: 5g

- Potassium: 130mg

- Phosphorus: 70mg

Serving Size: 1 glass

Cooking Time: 5 minutes

Preparation Time: 5 minutes

CHAPTER 7

Conclusion

Our goal in creating this Plant-Based Cookbook for CKD Stage 5 was to empower people living with Chronic Kidney Disease (CKD) to go on a culinary journey that not only meets their health needs but also thrills their taste senses. The recipes on these pages demonstrate how you can enjoy flavorful, fulfilling meals while sticking to the dietary limitations that come with CKD Stage 5.

Navigating the problems of CKD necessitates a comprehensive strategy, with nutrition playing a critical role in symptom management, minimizing complications, and improving overall wellness. The plant-based dishes offered here are not only kidney-friendly, but also aim to make each meal a celebration of different flavors, textures, and nutrient-dense ingredients.

From vivid smoothies to refreshing beverages, each dish is a carefully created combination of flavors, with potassium, phosphorus, and salt levels kept under control. The emphasis on complete, plant-based foods ensures that CKD Stage 5 nutritional requirements are addressed while maintaining taste.

As you embark on this culinary journey, we encourage you to see food as a source of healing and nourishment. Experiment with the recipes, make them your own, and enjoy the satisfaction of preparing meals that benefit your health. Remember that the route to better health entails not only limitation, but also embracing nature's cornucopia of nutrient-dense, delightful meals.

In addition to the recipes, consider making other lifestyle changes including staying hydrated, engaging in regular physical activity, and communicating openly with healthcare experts. Despite the obstacles of CKD Stage 5, the combination of a plant-based diet and a holistic approach to health can lead to a meaningful existence.

Finally, this cookbook serves as an empowerment tool, inspiring and guiding you to make informed and enjoyable nutritional choices. May each meal be a step toward greater health, and may your culinary journey be filled with pleasure, flavor, and vitality.

DAILY MEAL PLANNER

DAY/DATE: _______________________________

BREAKFAST

GROCERY LIST

LUNCH

DINNER

SNACKS

NOTES

DAILY MEAL PLANNER

DAY/DATE: _______________________________

BREAKFAST

GROCERY LIST

LUNCH

DINNER

SNACKS

NOTES

DAILY MEAL PLANNER

DAY/DATE: _______________________________

BREAKFAST

GROCERY LIST

LUNCH

DINNER

SNACKS

NOTES

DAILY MEAL PLANNER

DAY/DATE: _______________________________

BREAKFAST

GROCERY LIST

LUNCH

DINNER

SNACKS

NOTES

DAILY MEAL PLANNER

DAY/DATE: _______________________

BREAKFAST

GROCERY LIST

LUNCH

DINNER

SNACKS

NOTES

DAILY MEAL PLANNER

DAY/DATE: _______________________________

BREAKFAST

LUNCH

DINNER

SNACKS

GROCERY LIST

NOTES

DAILY MEAL PLANNER

DAY/DATE: _______________________________

BREAKFAST

GROCERY LIST

LUNCH

DINNER

SNACKS

NOTES

DAILY MEAL PLANNER

DAY/DATE: _______________________________

BREAKFAST

GROCERY LIST

LUNCH

DINNER

SNACKS

NOTES

DAILY MEAL PLANNER

DAY/DATE: _______________________________

BREAKFAST

GROCERY LIST

LUNCH

DINNER

SNACKS

NOTES

DAILY MEAL PLANNER

DAY/DATE: _______________________________

BREAKFAST

GROCERY LIST

LUNCH

DINNER

SNACKS

NOTES

DAILY MEAL PLANNER

DAY/DATE: _______________________________

BREAKFAST

GROCERY LIST

LUNCH

DINNER

SNACKS

NOTES

DAILY MEAL PLANNER

DAY/DATE: _______________________________

BREAKFAST

GROCERY LIST

LUNCH

DINNER

SNACKS

NOTES

DAILY MEAL PLANNER

DAY/DATE: _______________________________

BREAKFAST

LUNCH

DINNER

SNACKS

GROCERY LIST

NOTES

DAILY MEAL PLANNER

DAY/DATE: _______________________________

BREAKFAST

GROCERY LIST

LUNCH

DINNER

SNACKS

NOTES

DAILY MEAL PLANNER

DAY/DATE: _______________________________

BREAKFAST

GROCERY LIST

LUNCH

DINNER

SNACKS

NOTES

DAILY MEAL PLANNER

DAY/DATE: _______________________________

BREAKFAST

GROCERY LIST

LUNCH

DINNER

SNACKS

NOTES

DAILY MEAL PLANNER

DAY/DATE: _______________________________

BREAKFAST

GROCERY LIST

LUNCH

DINNER

SNACKS

NOTES

DAILY MEAL PLANNER

DAY/DATE: _________________________________

BREAKFAST

GROCERY LIST

LUNCH

DINNER

SNACKS

NOTES

DAILY MEAL PLANNER

DAY/DATE: _______________________________

BREAKFAST

GROCERY LIST

LUNCH

DINNER

SNACKS

NOTES

DAILY MEAL PLANNER

DAY/DATE: _______________________________

BREAKFAST

GROCERY LIST

LUNCH

DINNER

SNACKS

NOTES

DAILY MEAL PLANNER

DAY/DATE: _______________________________

BREAKFAST

GROCERY LIST

LUNCH

DINNER

SNACKS

NOTES

DAILY MEAL PLANNER

DAY/DATE: _______________________________

BREAKFAST

LUNCH

DINNER

GROCERY LIST

SNACKS

NOTES

DAILY MEAL PLANNER

DAY/DATE: _______________________________

BREAKFAST

GROCERY LIST

LUNCH

DINNER

SNACKS

NOTES

DAILY MEAL PLANNER

DAY/DATE: _______________________________

BREAKFAST

GROCERY LIST

LUNCH

DINNER

SNACKS

NOTES

DAILY MEAL PLANNER

DAY/DATE: _______________________________

| BREAKFAST | GROCERY LIST |

| LUNCH |

| DINNER |

| SNACKS | NOTES |

DAILY MEAL PLANNER

DAY/DATE: _______________________________

BREAKFAST

GROCERY LIST

LUNCH

DINNER

SNACKS

NOTES

DAILY MEAL PLANNER

DAY/DATE: _______________________________

BREAKFAST

GROCERY LIST

LUNCH

DINNER

SNACKS

NOTES

DAILY MEAL PLANNER

DAY/DATE: _______________________________

BREAKFAST

GROCERY LIST

LUNCH

DINNER

SNACKS

NOTES